A&L's QUICK REVIEW

PHARMACY

A&L's QUICK REVIEW

PHARMACY

12th edition

1000
Questions and Answers

Joyce A. Generali, MS, RPh, FASHP
Director, Drug Information Center
Pharmacy Department
Kansas University Medical Center
Kansas City, Kansas

Clinical Associate Professor
Department of Pharmacy Practice
University of Kansas
Lawrence, Kansas

Christine A. Berger, Pharm.D.
Director, Pharmacy Practice Experience Program
Clinical Assistant Professor
University of Kansas School of Pharmacy
Department of Pharmacy Practice
Lawrence, Kansas

Appleton & Lange Reviews/McGraw-Hill
Medical Publishing Division

New York Chicago San Francisco Lisbon London Madrid
Mexico City Milan New Delhi San Juan Seoul
Singapore Sydney Toronto

McGraw-Hill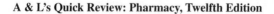

A Division of The McGraw-Hill Companies

A & L's Quick Review: Pharmacy, Twelfth Edition

2 3 4 5 6 7 8 9 0   DOC/DOC   0 9 8 7 6 5 4

ISBN 0-07-140220-9 (Domestic)
ISBN 0-07-137747-6 (Domestic Set)
ISBN 0-07-140221-7 (Domestic CD)

This book was set in Times Roman by North Market Street Graphics.
The editors were Patricia Casey, Catherine A. Johnson, and Karen Davis.
The production supervisor was Richard Ruzycka.
The cover designer was Mary McKeon.
R.R. Donnelley & Sons, Crawfordsville, was printer and binder.

This book is printed on acid-free paper.

Library of Congress Cataloging-in-Publication Data
Generali, Joyce A.
    Pharmacy : 985 questions & answers / Joyce A. Generali, Christine A.
      Berger.— 12th ed.
      p.; cm. — (Appleton and Lange's quick review)
    Includes bibliographical references.
    ISBN 0-07-137747-6 (alk. paper)
    1. Pharmacy—Examinations, questions, etc.   2. Pharmacology—
Examinations, questions, etc.   I. Berger, Christine A.   II. Title.
III. A & L's quick review.
    [DNLM: 1. Pharmacology—Examination Questions. QV 18.2 G326a 2002]
RS97 .G47 2002
615'.1'076—dc21

                              2002025491

ISBN 0-07-121315-5 (International)
ISBN 0-07-121241-8 (International Set)
ISBN 0-07-121316-3 (International CD)

Exclusive rights by The McGraw-Hill Companies, Inc., for manufacture and export. This book cannot be re-exported from the country to which it is consigned by McGraw-Hill. The International Edition is not available in North America.

This book is dedicated to our families:

To our children Matthew, Scott, Jessica, and Jonathan.

And to our husbands Steven and Ron for their support and encouragement of our personal and professional endeavors.

A special thanks to my father S.D. Generali, whose encouragement has been unwavering and in memorial to my mother Vilma E. Generali, whose grace and spirit remain with me always.

Contents

Preface

NAPLEX, the North American Pharmacist Licensure Examination, is designed to test the knowledge considered necessary for entry level pharmacists, regardless of practice setting. It is an examination, which consists of 185 multiple-choice questions. However, only 150 of these are used to calculate the final score. The remaining 35 questions are pretest questions which are being evaluated for future exams.

Quick Review: 12th Edition provides pharmacy students the opportunity to test their knowledge in all the major areas of pharmacy study and to practice answering questions representative of the type and formats found on the actual NAPLEX.

The book is divided into six chapters. The first five chapters provide questions and explanatory answers on the major topics of a pharmacy school curriculum: Pharmaceutics/Pharmacokinetics, Pharmacology, Microbiology and Public Health, Biochemistry and Chemistry, and Physiology and Pathology. By testing their knowledge of these topics, pharmacy students can quickly identify their strengths and weaknesses and decide where added emphasis is needed in preparation for the examination.

A majority of the questions on the NAPLEX are scenario based (i.e., a patient case with accompanying questions). Chapter 6, Clinical Pharmacy, is a compilation of questions that refer to patient profiles or prescriptions, similar to the format found on NAPLEX. In answering these questions, students are expected to apply factual knowledge to a practical situation. This chapter is similar in format to NAPLEX and can be used as a practice test.

The multiple-choice questions in all six chapters are written in the stylistic convention of the NAPLEX. Answers and discussion follow each chapter. Students are advised to read *each* question carefully. Negative statements, such as **NOT, NEVER,** and **EXCEPT,** are capitalized and printed in bold face to help the student focus on the correct approach to the question. The questions are based on the NAPLEX Competency Statements. These competency statements can be found at the following website:

http://www.nabp.net/index.asp?target=/whatsnew/newsletters/1999-10/article5.asp&

Also we recommend consulting the latest edition of *NAPLEX: A Candidate's Review Guide.*

In utilizing this review book, students are encouraged to use deductive reasoning in selecting responses to each question instead of attempting to memorize individual facts. The student thereby improves his or her test-taking skills with multiple choice examinations while enhancing his or her knowledge of critical pharmacy information.

In 1997, NAPLEX adopted a computer adaptive (CAT) approach to testing. This method individualized the exam to each candidate's level of ability based on responses to previous questions. On the CD-ROM provided with this product you will have the ability to refer to previous questions in order to optimize studying. However, during the testing mode, the CD-ROM will simulate the NAPLEX so that you will be unable to omit or skip a question and you cannot review questions already answered. The study CD-ROM includes the following key features:

- Ability to create multiple customized practice tests
- Save comments in an electronic notebook while studying
- Provide assessment of strengths and weaknesses
- Digital time to show elapsed study time

Review Tips

Common Conversions

Memorizing these standard concentrations will make conversions easier.

- There is 1 mg of epinephrine in 1 mL of a 1:1000 solution.
- There are 40 mEq of potassium in 30 mL of a 10% potassium chloride solution.
- An 8.4% solution of sodium bicarbonate contains 1 mEq each of sodium and bicarbonate ions per mL.
- There are 154 mEq of sodium in 1000 mL of 0.9% sodium chloride.
- There are 50 grams of dextrose in 1000 mL of D5W.
- There are 1700 calories in 1000 ml of D50W (500 grams of dextrose).
- 400,000 units of penicillin are equivalent to 250 mg.
- A nitroglycerin 0.4 mg sublingual tablet contains 1/150 grains.

Miscellaneous Review Lists

The following lists are intended to provide a brief review. They are by no means comprehensive and should not be used to make medical recommendations.

Transdermal Systems Should Be Changed Accordingly

Clonidine patch	every 7 days
Estradiol patch	once–twice weekly (depending on brand of product)
Fentanyl patch	every 3 days
Nicotine patch	every day

| Nitroglycerin patch | every day |
| Scopolamine patch | every 3 days |

Common Vitamins and the Condition That Results From Their Deficiency

Ascorbic acid (vitamin C)	Scurvy
Cyanocobalamin (vitamin B_{12})	Pernicious anemia
Folic acid	Megaloblastic anemia
Niacin (nicotinic acid)	Pellagra
Thiamine (vitamin B_1)	Beriberi, Wernicke-Korsakoff syndrome
Vitamin D	Rickets

Viruses and Antiviral Agents That Inhibit Them

Cytomegalovirus	Cidofovir (Vistide)
	Ganciclovir (Cytovene)
	Foscarnet (Foscavir)
	Fomivirsen (Vitravene)
Hepatitis B virus	Interferon alfa-2b (Intron A)
	Lamivudine (Epivir HBV)
Herpes simplex virus	Acyclovir (Zovirax)
	Famciclovir (Famvir)
	Valacyclovir (Valtrex)
Influenza A virus	Amantadine (Symmetrel)
	Rimantadine (Flumadine)
Influenza A and B virus	Oseltamivir (Tamiflu)
	Zanamivir (Relenza)
Respiratory syncytial virus	Ribavirin (Rebetron)
Varicella-zoster virus	Acyclovir (Zovirax)
	Famciclovir (Famvir)
	Valacyclovir (Valtrex)

Medications and Their Antidotes

Acetaminophen	Acetylcysteine
Benzodiazepines	Flumazenil

Digoxin	Digoxin immune fab
Dopamine	Phentolamine
Heparin	Protamine
Iron	Deferoxamine
Methotrexate	Leucovorin
Morphine (opiates)	Naloxone
Nitrogen mustard	Sodium thiosulfate
Organophosphates	Pralidoxime/2-PAM
Warfarin	Phytonadione/vitamin K

Laboratory Tests and What They Indicate

ANA titer	Rheumatic diseases
aPTT	Monitor heparin therapy
Coombs	Antibody screening for blood donor/recipient compatibility
D-xylose	GI function
Guaiac	Occult blood in the stool
INR	Monitor warfarin therapy
Prothrombin time	Monitor warfarin therapy
Reinsch	Screen for heavy metals
Schillings	Vitamin B_{12} absorption (pernicious anemia)
Sweat test	Cystic fibrosis

Drugs Commonly Associated With Hepatic Failure

Acetaminophen	Ketoconazole
Alcohol	L-asparaginase
Allopurinol	Methotrexate
Carbamazepine	Niacin
Cytarabine	Oral contraceptives
Erythromycin (estolate salt)	Parenteral nutrition
Flucytosine	Rifampin
Gancyclovir	Sulfonylureas
Isoniazid	Valproate

Drugs Commonly Associated With Decreased Renal Function

Aminoglycosides   Cyclosporine
Amphotericin B   Foscarnet
Cisplatin   Pentamidine

Drugs Associated With Folic Acid Deficiency Anemia

Barbiturates   Primidone
Methotrexate   Pyrimethamine
Oral contraceptives   Sulfasalazine
Phenytoin   Trimethoprim

Drugs Associated With Lupus Erythematosus-like Reaction

Ethosuximide   Phenothiazines
Hydralazine   Phenytoin
Isoniazid   Procainamide
Methyldopa   Quinidine
Nitrofurantoin   Sulfonamides
Penicillamine   Tetracyclines

Drugs Associated With Pancreatitis

Alcohol   Metronidazole
L-asparaginase   Parenteral nutrition
Azathioprine   Pentamidine
Cimetidine   Ranitidine
Dideoxyinosine (DDI)   Sulfonamides
Estrogens   Tetracycline
Furosemide   Thiazides
Glucocorticoids   Valproate
Mercaptopurine

Drugs Associated With Photosensitivity Reactions

Amiodarone
Amitriptyline
Doxepine
Fluoxetine
Furosemide
Griseofulvin
Isotretinoin
Ketoprofen
Nalidixic acid

Naproxen
Oral contraceptives
Oral hypoglycemics
Phenothiazines
Piroxicam
Sulfonamides
Tetracycline
Thiazides

Drug-induced Parkinson's Disease May Be Caused by

Butyrophenones (especially haloperidol)
Heavy metal poisoning

Phenothiazines (especially thorazine)
Reserpine

Drugs Associated With Hyperglycemia

Amiodarone
L-asparaginase
Epinephrine
Estrogens
Glucocorticoids
Lithium

Nicotinic acid
Oral contraceptives
Pentamidine
Phenytoin
Thyroid hormones

Drugs to Avoid in Pregnancy

Atorvastatin
Benzodiazepines
Ergotamine
Finasteride
Fluorouracil
Fluoroquinolones
Fluvastatin
Hormonal agents
Isotretinoin
Lovastatin

Methotrexate
Misoprostol
Pravastatin
Raloxifene
Simvastatin
Tetracyclines
Thalidomide
Vitamin A palmitate
Warfarin

Drugs That Should Not Be Taken With Food

Ampicillin	Labetalol
Astemizole	Lansoprazole
Cefaclor	Levodopa
Didanosine	Lithium
Digoxin	Metoprolol
Diltiazem	Nimodipine
Etidronate	Penicillamine
Furosemide	Propranolol
Indinavir	Rifampin
Isoniazid	Zafirlukast

Medications That Should Not Be Administered With Antacids

Digoxin	Quinidine
Fluoroquinolones	Tetracycline
Isoniazid	Warfarin
Ketoconazole	

Common Emulsifying Agents Used in Pharmaceuticals Include

Acacia	Pectin
Agar	Sodium lauryl sulfate
Gelatin	Tragacanth
Methylcellulose	

Common Preservatives Used in Pharmaceuticals Include

Benzalkonium chloride	Phenylmercuric acetate
Benzyl alcohol	Potassium sorbate
Boric acid	Propylparaben
Chlorobutanol	Sodium bisulfite
Disodium edetate	Sodium borate
Methylparaben	Thimersol
Phenol	

Common Suspending Agents Used in Pharmaceuticals Include

Alginic acid	Sodium carboxymethyl-cellulose
Carrageenin	

Common Pharmaceutical Substances and Their USP Names

Burow's solution	Aluminum acetate solution (an astringent)
Dakin's solution	Sodium hypochlorite solution (diluted bleach)
Lime water	Calcium hydroxide solution
Sweet oil	Olive oil

Drugs That Are Highly Protein Bound

Barbiturates	Sulfur/sulfonamides
Clofibrate	Tolbutamide
Salicylates	Warfarin

Agents That Inhibit the P-450 Microsomal Enzyme System

Allopurinol	Metronidazole
Anabolic agents	Monoamine oxidase inhibitors
Chloramphenicol	
Cimetidine	Oral antidiabetic agents
Disulfiram	Warfarin
Isoniazid	

Agents That Induce the P-450 Microsomal Enzyme System

Alcohol	Nicotine
Chloral hydrate	Phenobarbital
Chlordiazepoxide	Phenytoin
Cortisone	Prednisone
Imipramine	Testosterone

OTC Cough and Cold Products Commonly Contain the Following

Analgesic	Acetaminophen
Antihistamine	Brompheniramine

	Chlorpheniramine
	Clemastine
	Diphenhydramine
	Pyrilamine
	Triprolidine
Cough suppressant	Codeine
	Dextromethorphan
Decongestant	Phenylephrine
	Phenylpropanolamine
	Pseudoephedrine
Expectorant	Ammonium chloride
	Guaifenesin
	Sodium citrate

Pharmaceutical References and What They Contain

AHFS Drug Information (American Hospital Formulary Service)	Displays the structure of each of the drugs referenced
Merck Manual	List of diseases and how to treat
Merck Index	Encyclopedia of chemicals, drugs, and biologicals
Red Book	Prices, lists of sugar-free, alcohol-free products, pregnancy categories, photosensitivity information, etc.
Remington's	Compounding information

Normal Lab Values of Electrolytes and Minerals

Sodium	135–147 mEq/L
Potassium	3.5–5.0 mEq/L
Chloride	95–105 mEq/L
Magnesium	1.5–2.2 mEq/L
Calcium	8.5–10.8 mg/dL
Phosphate	2.6–4.5 mg/dL

PHARMACY

1

Pharmaceutics/ Pharmacokinetics

DIRECTIONS (Questions 1–150): Each of the questions or incomplete statements below is followed by five suggested answers or completions. Select the **one answer** that is best in each case.

1. Emulsions made with tweens are usually
   A. unstable
   B. w/o
   C. o/w
   D. clear
   E. reversible

2. Which of the following factors affect the distribution of a drug?
   A. Lipid solubility
   B. Plasma protein binding
   C. Polarity
   D. Molecular size
   E. All of the above

3. The rate of zero-order reactions
   A. changes constantly
   B. is independent of temperature
   C. is independent of concentration
   D. holds only for light-catalyzed reactions
   E. holds only for radioactive compounds

4. Spans and tweens are
   A. highly polymerized mannuronic acid anhydrides
   B. phospholipids
   C. polyoxyalkalene derivatives
   D. glycosides
   E. none of the above

5. Lidocaine HC1 is **NOT** administered orally because it is
   A. ineffective by this route
   B. too acidic
   C. too toxic by this route
   D. a cause of arrhythmias
   E. unstable

6. The two major properties of drugs that are usually modified
   by complexation are
   A. odor and taste
   B. taste and solubility
   C. chemical structure and solubility
   D. chemical structure and stability
   E. stability and solubility

7. What will result if the distribution of drugs is slower than the
   processes of biotransformation and elimination?
   A. High blood levels of drug
   B. Low blood levels of drug
   C. Synergism
   D. Potentiation
   E. Failure to attain diffusion equilibrium

8. In radiopharmacy, the term "rem" means
   A. radiations per millisecond
   B. radiations per minute
   C. roentgen-equivalent-man
   D. external roentgens per minute
   E. roentgen exposure per minute

9. pH is
   A. not temperature dependent
   B. a measure of acidity
   C. the same as pOH

D. high for acids
E. none of the above

10. Which of the following types of tissues frequently stores drugs?
    A. Fatty tissue
    B. Muscle tissue
    C. Protein tissue
    D. A and B
    E. A and C

11. Which of the following drugs undergoes marked hydrolysis in the GI tract?
    A. Aspirin
    B. Penicillin G
    C. Acetaminophen
    D. Hydrocortisone
    E. Chlortetracycline

12. Precipitated sulfur is often incorporated into ointments to be used as a
    A. parasiticide (e.g., for scabies)
    B. emollient
    C. keratolytic
    D. A and C only
    E. A, B, and C

13. Solutions that contain bacteriostatic agents
    A. cannot be tested for sterility
    B. must be cultured on agar plates for sterility tests
    C. must be diluted beyond the bacteriostatic level for sterility tests
    D. do not require a sterility test
    E. are none of the above

14. A source of anticarcinogenic drugs is
    A. belladonna
    B. nux vomica
    C. vinca rosea
    D. cascara
    E. digitalis

15. If a central nervous system (CNS) drug is extensively ion-
    ized at the pH of blood, it will
    A. penetrate the blood–brain barrier slowly
    B. penetrate the blood–brain barrier rapidly
    C. not penetrate the blood–brain barrier
    D. be eliminated slowly
    E. not be distributed to any tissue sites

16. Pharmacists should caution patients who are taking niacin
    that this drug
    A. stains the urine bright red
    B. causes ringing in the ears
    C. causes muscular weakness
    D. should be taken before meals
    E. should be taken with meals

17. If a drug has a biological half-life of 6.9 days, the best dos-
    ing interval would be
    A. weekly
    B. biweekly
    C. semiweekly
    D. qid
    E. daily

18. First-order half-life is equal to
    A. 1/k
    B. k
    C. 0.693/k
    D. 2k + 1
    E. none of the above

19. A prescription calls for 25 mg of potassium chloride. How
    many grams of KCl (MW 74.6) are needed?
    A. 7.46 g
    B. 0.746 g
    C. 8.86 g
    D. 1.86 g
    E. 0.186 g

20. An IV order requires 5 million units of sodium penicillin G to be added to 1 L of normal saline. How many mEq of sodium are available per liter of solution?
    A. 154.0 mEq
    B. 1540.0 mEq
    C. 8.4 mEq
    D. 162.0 mEq
    E. 1620.0 mEq

21. An order calls for 500 cc of a solution of potassium sulfate to be made so that it contains 10 mEq of K^+. How many grams of potassium sulfate are required?
    A. 0.440 g
    B. 4.440 g
    C. 0.044 g
    D. 0.870 g
    E. 8.700 g

22. How many milliliters of a 10% KCl (MW 74.6) solution contain 5.0 mEq of K^+?
    A. 2.100 mL
    B. 21.000 mL
    C. 3.730 mL
    D. 37.300 mL
    E. 0.373 mL

23. One hundred milligrams (100 mg) of a drug are given as an IV bolus. The drug fits a one-compartment, first-order pharmacokinetic model. The volume of distribution is 20 L. The plasma concentration immediately after administration (at time 0) is
    A. 20 mg/L
    B. 10 mg/cc
    C. 2 mg/cc
    D. 15 mg/cc
    E. 5 mg/L

24. Most drugs are
   A. strong electrolytes
   B. weak electrolytes
   C. nonelectrolytes
   D. highly ionic
   E. none of the above

25. The major mechanism of degradation of drugs in the GI tract is
   A. oxidation
   B. hydrolysis
   C. acetylation
   D. conjugation
   E. reduction

26. The buffer equation is also known as
   A. Young's equation
   B. Charles' law
   C. Henderson–Hasselbalch equation
   D. Stokes' law
   E. none of the above

27. The pKw of water at 25°C is
   A. 7
   B. 14
   C. 1×10^{-14}
   D. 1×10^{-7}
   E. 1

28. Which of the following is **NOT** a major pathway or type of biotransformation?
   A. Oxidation
   B. Deamination
   C. Reduction
   D. Hydrolysis
   E. Conjugation

29. When making pharmacokinetic recommendations in aminoglycoside dosing, if you want to decrease only the trough concentration, you would
   A. decrease the dose
   B. take the trough measurement 3 hours before the next dose

C. lengthen the dosing interval
D. increase the dose
E. none of the above

30. The dose of a drug is 0.5 mg/kg. What dose should be given a 6-year-old child who weighs 44 lb?
    A. 0.003 g
    B. 0.033 g
    C. 0.010 g
    D. 0.100 g
    E. 0.050 g

31. If a prescription order requires 30 g of concentrated sulfuric acid (density is 1.8 g/mL), what volume should the pharmacist measure?
    A. 1.67 mL
    B. 18.00 mL
    C. 30.00 mL
    D. 16.67 mL
    E. 166.70 mL

32. Calculate the weight of 25 mL of hydrochloric acid whose density is 1.18 g/mL.
    A. 29.500 g
    B. 2.950 g
    C. 0.295 g
    D. 295.00 g
    E. None of the above

33. In most biotransformation reactions, the metabolite of a drug
    A. is more polar than the parent compound
    B. is more lipid soluble than the parent compound
    C. has a longer $t_{1/2}$ than the parent compound
    D. is all of the above
    E. is none of the above

34. To calculate a loading dose, one must first determine
    A. $t_{1/2}$
    B. body clearance
    C. fraction protein bound
    D. volume of distribution
    E. all of the above

35. Convert 60 grams to grains
    A. 9240 grains
    B. 924 grains
    C. 9.24 grains
    D. 0.924 grains
    E. 0.0924 grains

36. Radioactive decay follows a
    A. mixed-order rate
    B. fractional-order rate
    C. zero-order rate
    D. first-order rate
    E. second-order rate

37. The HLB system is used to classify
    A. flavors
    B. colors
    C. surfactants
    D. organic ring structures
    E. perfumes

38. Alpha particles are very similar to
    A. hydrogen atoms
    B. helium atoms
    C. neutrons
    D. protons
    E. electrons

39. To achieve the same steady-state plasma concentration (for a drug that is excreted by the kidney) in renal failure patients as in patients with normal renal function, you should
    A. increase the dosing interval
    B. decrease the dose
    C. adjust both the dose and the dosing interval
    D. do any of the above, depending on the pharmacodynamic properties of the drug
    E. not adjust the dosing regimen unless the patient shows signs of toxicity

40. The most common disintegrator in compressed tablets is
 A. dextrose
 B. lactose
 C. starch
 D. potassium bitartrate
 E. powdered sucrose

41. Freons are
 A. alkanes
 B. alkenes
 C. alkynes
 D. fluorinated hydrocarbons
 E. a mixture of CO_2 and air

42. Which of the following factors may make it necessary to give lower doses of drugs to geriatric patients?
 A. Reduced enzyme activity
 B. Reduced kidney function
 C. Enhanced absorption
 D. A and B only
 E. A, B, and C

43. Convert 2 pints 3 fluid ounces into mL.
 A. 1500 mL
 B. 1050 mL
 C. 150 mL
 D. 105 mL
 E. 10.5 mL

44. Tablet hardness range is normally
 A. 0.2 to 0.5 kg
 B. 0.5 to 1.0 kg
 C. 1.0 to 2.0 kg
 D. 2.0 to 3.5 kg
 E. 3.5 to 7.0 kg

45. An antidote for heparin overdosage is
 A. protamine sulfate
 B. BAL
 C. atropine
 D. calcium salts
 E. dicumarol

46. The dose of a drug is 0.6 mg. How many doses are contained in 96 mg of the drug?
   A. 16
   B. 160
   C. 360
   D. 600
   E. None of the above

47. Which of the following may be used as plasma expanders?
   A. Sodium salts
   B. Dextrans
   C. Starches
   D. Calcium salts
   E. Prostaglandins

48. The expression "ppm" as used in compounding prescriptions most often is defined as
   A. parts per million
   B. parts per mL
   C. parts per mole
   D. pieces per million
   E. parts per molar

49. GMP regulations (USFDA) primarily apply to
   A. controlled drugs
   B. wholesalers
   C. pharmaceutical manufacturers
   D. hospital pharmacy
   E. community pharmacy

50. pH is equivalent to pka at
   A. pH of 7
   B. pH of 1
   C. pH of 14
   D. half neutralization point
   E. neutralization point

51. A popular theory of acids and bases is
   A. Boyle's law
   B. Four Humors' theory
   C. Pythagorean theory

D. Bronsted–Lowry theory
E. Henry's theory

52. Salicylic acid is used primarily as a (an)
  A. analgesic
  B. antipyretic
  C. cough suppressant
  D. uricosuric agent
  E. keratolytic agent

53. Pyridoxine is
  A. vitamin B_6
  B. vitamin A
  C. vitamin B_1
  D. vitamin K
  E. vitamin D

54. Glycerin has a specific gravity of 1.25. One gallon weighs
  A. 591.25 g
  B. 473.0 g
  C. 4730.0 g
  D. 128.0 g
  E. 4800.0 g

55. Vitamin K is associated with
  A. pellagra
  B. nerves
  C. hemoglobin concentration
  D. bones
  E. blood clotting

56. Which of the following is found in vitamin B_{12}?
  A. Magnesium
  B. Nickel
  C. Iron
  D. Cobalt
  E. Manganese

57. Another name for polyethylene glycol polymers is
  A. sodium alginate
  B. silica gel
  C. Carbowax
  D. Friar paste
  E. none of the above

58. $-12°C$ is equivalent to
  A. 36.0°F
  B. 12.0°F
  C. 10.4°F
  D. 5.0°F
  E. -2°F

59. One tablespoon is approximately equivalent to
  A. 15 mL
  B. 10 mL
  C. 8 mL
  D. 20 mL
  E. 30 mL

60. When describing solubility terms, >10,000 parts of solvent for 1 part of solute would be called
  A. very soluble
  B. soluble
  C. sparingly soluble
  D. slightly soluble
  E. practically insoluble or insoluble

61. The amount of 190 proof required to make 500 cc of 70% alcohol is
  A. 350 cc
  B. 520 cc
  C. 184 cc
  D. 368 cc
  E. 37 cc

62. Which of the following dose forms is specifically covered by the Federal Hazardous Substance Labeling Act?
  A. Parenterals
  B. Aerosols

C. Tinctures
D. Ophthalmic solutions
E. Nitroglycerin tablets

63. Which of the following ions plays a significant role in preventing convulsions?
A. Potassium
B. Lithium
C. Magnesium
D. Sodium
E. Fluoride

64. The chemical substance used commonly in running a GI series is
A. barium sulfate
B. fluorescein dye
C. radioactive iodine
D. sodium bicarbonate
E. sodium carbonate

65. Colleges of pharmacy are accredited by
A. the AFPE
B. the AACP
C. the ACPE
D. the NABP
E. none of the above

66. Denaturation of emulsions is characterized by
A. irreversible precipitation
B. reversible precipitation
C. creaming
D. changing of external phase
E. C and D

67. Characteristics of pyrogens include the following.
   I. They usually cause a febrile reaction in humans
   II. They may cause pains in the back and legs
   III. They may cause chills

   A. I only
   B. III only
   C. I and II only
   D. I and III only
   E. I, II, and III

68. Freeze drying is based on
   A. pressure filtration
   B. sublimation
   C. polymerization
   D. pasteurization
   E. densification

69. Lubricants in tablets serve the following functions.
   I. They improve the flow of tablet granulation
   II. They prevent adhesion to dies and punches
   III. They facilitate ejection from die cavity

   A. I only
   B. II only
   C. I and II only
   D. I and III only
   E. I, II, and III

70. The most prevalent commercial solid dosage forms are
   A. hard capsules
   B. soft gelatin capsules
   C. tablets
   D. bulk powders
   E. divided powders

71. Which of the following is **NOT** a naturally occurring emulsifier?
   A. Acacia
   B. Cholesterol
   C. Gelatin

D. Veegum
E. Tragacanth

72. The purpose of sorbitol in formulations of soft gelatin capsules is as a (an)
    A. plasticizer
    B. disintegrating agent
    C. lubricant
    D. thickener
    E. emulsifier

73. Hard gelatin capsules for human use are available in the following sizes.
    I. 1
    II. 00
    III. 0000

    A. I only
    B. II only
    C. III only
    D. I and II only
    E. I, II, and III

74. Ointments are typically used as
    I. emollients
    II. protective barriers
    III. vehicles for applying drugs

    A. I only
    B. III only
    C. I and II only
    D. II and III only
    E. I, II, and III

75. A humectant retards
    A. bacterial growth
    B. degradation
    C. surface evaporation
    D. spreadability
    E. all of the above

76. The Noyes–Whitney equation describes
  A. zero-order kinetics
  B. first-order kinetics
  C. mixed-order kinetics
  D. dissolution rate
  E. renal clearance

77. Starch is used in tabletting as a
  I. binder
  II. glidant
  III. disintegrant

  A. II only
  B. III only
  C. I and II only
  D. II and III only
  E. I, II, and III

78. Which of the following properties is characteristic of flocculated particles in suspension?
  A. particles form loose aggregates
  B. rate of sedimentation is high
  C. a sediment is formed rapidly
  D. the sediment is loosely packed
  E. all of the above

79. Gums are used in tabletting primarily as
  A. disintegrators
  B. glidants
  C. lubricants
  D. binding agents
  E. both B and C

80. Which of the following is (are) true for buccal and sublingual tablets?
  I. They are useful for drugs destroyed by gastric fluid
  II. They are readily soluble
  III. They are useful for drugs that are poorly absorbed in the intestinal tract

A. I and II only
B. II and III only
C. II only
D. III only
E. I, II, and III

81. Vanishing creams are classified as
A. oleaginous
B. absorption bases
C. water-soluble bases
D. o/w bases
E. w/o bases

82. Syrup NF is
A. self-preserving
B. a supersaturated solution
C. a dilute solution
D. highly unstable
E. flavored and preserved

83. Which of the following would be classified as a strong acid according to acid–base theory?
A. 10% acetic acid
B. 5% boric acid
C. 0.5% hydrochloric acid
D. 100% oleic acid
E. None because all are weak acids

84. Reaction rate is increased most readily by
A. humidity
B. high temperature
C. freezing
D. photolysis
E. hydrolysis

85. Dissolution rate is increased by
  I. an increase in surface area
  II. a decrease in particle size
  III. the formation of molecular aggregates

  A. I only
  B. II only
  C. II and III only
  D. I and II only
  E. I, II, and III

86. Units for renal clearance are in
  A. mg/L
  B. g/L
  C. cc/min
  D. mg%
  E. all of the above

87. GMP regulations are promulgated and revised by
  A. Congress
  B. state boards of pharmacy
  C. the DEA
  D. the FDA
  E. the EPA

88. A primary disadvantage of ethylene glycol as a solvent in oral preparations is its
  A. potential toxicity
  B. lack of solvent action
  C. very limited miscibility
  D. high cost
  E. high viscosity

89. Glucose is **NOT** subject to hydrolysis because it is
  A. a disaccharide
  B. a monosaccharide
  C. a polysaccharide
  D. insoluble
  E. both B and C

90. Purified water USP may **NOT** be used in
   A. syrups
   B. topical preparations
   C. parenteral preparations
   D. elixirs
   E. effervescent solutions

91. Ferritin is a (an)
   A. vitamin
   B. micelle
   C. emulsion
   D. amino acid
   E. protein

92. Vitamin B_6 is also known as
   A. thiamine
   B. riboflavin
   C. niacin
   D. pyridoxine
   E. cyanocobalamin

93. HLB is a system used to distinguish between
   A. surfactants
   B. glidants
   C. suspending agents
   D. excipients
   E. disintegrators

94. Disadvantages of chlorobutanol in germicide solutions include
   I. heat instability
   II. instability at alkaline pH
   III. loss of potency in presence of air

   A. I only
   B. II only
   C. I and II only
   D. I, II, and III
   E. II and III only

95. A solution has an osmolal concentration of one when it contains
   A. 1 osmol of solute/kg of water
   B. 1 osmol of solute/mL of water
   C. 1 osmol of solute/L water
   D. 1 osmol of solute/kg of sodium chloride
   E. 1 osmol of solute/mL of sodium chloride

96. Sunscreen preparations containing *p*-aminobenzoic acid should be
   A. used sparingly
   B. applied 2 hours before exposure
   C. packaged in air-tight containers
   D. packaged in light-resistant containers
   E. used only on areas other than the face

97. Which of the following statements is (are) true for undecylenic acid?
   I. It is often used as the zinc salt
   II. It may cause irritation and sensitization
   III. It is the most fungistatic of the fatty acids

   A. I only
   B. I and II only
   C. II only
   D. I and III only
   E. I, II, and III

98. Which of the following is classified as fat soluble?
   A. Vitamin D
   B. Niacin
   C. Ascorbic acid
   D. Thiamine hydrochloride
   E. Riboflavin

99. The active constituents of saline laxatives are
   A. absorbable anions
   B. nonabsorbable cations
   C. tribasic cations
   D. absorbable cations and anions
   E. nonabsorbable cations and anions

100. Bismuth subsalicylate is used in antidiarrheals for its
   A. hydrophobic action
   B. hydrophilic action
   C. adsorbent action
   D. absorbent action
   E. antibacterial action

101. Sublimation is the term applied to the following type(s) of transformation.
   I. Solid to vapor
   II. Liquid to solid
   III. Liquid to vapor

   A. I only
   B. II only
   C. III only
   D. I and II only
   E. II and III only

102. Which of the following is a cationic emulsifying agent?
   A. Potassium laurate
   B. Calcium oleate
   C. Sodium lauryl sulfate
   D. Cetyltrimethylammonium bromide
   E. Ammonium laurate

103. Mineral oil exerts laxative action primarily by
   A. bulk formation
   B. fecal softening
   C. catharsis
   D. stimulation
   E. lubrication

104. Cellulose acetate phthalate is used in pharmacy as a (an)
   A. emulsifier
   B. enteric coating material
   C. suspending agent
   D. flavoring agent
   E. excipient

105. Cocoa butter (theobroma oil) is useful as a suppository base because of its
    A. solubility
    B. melting point
    C. miscibility
    D. reactivity
    E. lipophilic properties

106. The most widely used method for sterilization of pharmaceuticals is
    A. microfiltration
    B. radiation
    C. ethylene oxide exposure
    D. moist heat
    E. dry heat

107. Ophthalmic solutions should be formulated to include which of the following?
    I. Sterility
    II. Isotonicity
    III. Buffering

    A. I only
    B. II only
    C. I and II only
    D. II and III only
    E. I, II, and III

108. One form of the buffer equation is pH = pKa + log salt/acid. For this equation, the salt and acid concentration is expressed in
    A. g/100 cc
    B. moles
    C. mg %
    D. g/L
    E. none of the above

109. If a buffer solution is prepared using equal concentrations of acetic acid and sodium acetate, the pH would then be
    A. 1
    B. 14

C. equal to the pKa
D. equal to 1/2 of the pKa
E. equal to double the pKa

110. Another name for the buffer equation is the
    A. Arrhenius equation
    B. Henderson–Hasselbalch equation
    C. Debye–Huckel equation
    D. buffer capacity equation
    E. Stokes' equation

111. Which of the following is an ampholyte?
    A. H_2CO_3
    B. HCl
    C. NaOH
    D. NaH_2PO_4
    E. KOH

112. Soda lime is used as a (an)
    A. alkalinizer
    B. therapeutic agent in topical preparations
    C. stabilizer in emulsions
    D. reagent for absorption of carbon dioxide
    E. preservative in aromatic waters

113. Pumice is often used in
    I. soaps and cleansing powders
    II. dental preparation
    III. filtering

    A. I only
    B. II only
    C. III only
    D. I and III only
    E. I, II, and III

114. There was no requirement to establish efficacy for drug products until
   A. 1906
   B. 1938
   C. 1962
   D. 1965
   E. 1978

115. The type of instability known as "bleeding" is usually associated with
   A. isotonic solutions
   B. emulsions
   C. alcoholic solutions
   D. ointments
   E. suspensions

116. The GMP regulations first became official in
   A. 1938
   B. 1962
   C. 1963
   D. 1979
   E. 1981

117. The Limulus test is a relatively new method of testing for
   A. pyrogens
   B. microbial growth
   C. acidity
   D. creaming
   E. lack of osmolarity

118. Which of the following is associated with excessive infusion of hypotonic fluids?
   A. Hemolysis
   B. Hyperglycemia
   C. Dehydration
   D. Glycosuria
   E. None of the above

119. Which of the following is associated with excessive infusion of hypertonic dextrose solutions?
  A. Loss of electrolytes
  B. Hyperglycemia
  C. Dehydration
  D. Glycosuria
  E. All of the above

120. Normal rectal temperature is usually
  A. measured in the morning
  B. measured in the evening
  C. about the same as the normal oral temperature
  D. about 1° lower than oral
  E. about 1° higher than oral

121. The Latin *oculo utro* is translated to mean
  A. right eye
  B. each eye
  C. left eye
  D. each ear
  E. right ear

122. Advantages of tablets over liquid dose forms include the following.
  I. Enhanced stability
  II. Ease of administration
  III. Greater accuracy of dosing

  A. II only
  B. III only
  C. I and II only
  D. II and III only
  E. I, II, and III

123. Which of the following is (are) exempted from safety packaging?
    I. Oral contraceptives
    II. Nitroglycerin
    III. Oral analgesics

    A. I only
    B. II only
    C. I and II only
    D. II and III only
    E. I, II, and III

124. The Latin *post cibos* can be translated to mean
    A. after meals
    B. before meals
    C. with meals
    D. without food
    E. on an empty stomach

125. A disadvantage of using compressed gases in aerosol preparations is that they
    A. produce higher pressures
    B. produce incompatibilities
    C. contribute to instability
    D. produce a wet spray
    E. produce increased clogging

126. Prednisone is converted to which of the following by the liver?
    A. Cortisone
    B. Hydrocortisone
    C. Prednisolone
    D. Methylprednisolone
    E. Dexamethasone

127. Which of the following is (are) true for water-soluble vitamins?
    I. They have limited storage in the body
    II. They may be toxic in doses above MDR
    III. Most are eliminated by the kidneys

A. I only
B. II only
C. III only
D. I and II only
E. I, II, and III

128. The dose of a drug is 5 mg/kg body weight. What dose should be given to a 110-lb female patient?
A. 2500 mg
B. 250 mg
C. 25 mg
D. 44 mg
E. 440 mg

129. How many grains of a drug are needed to make 4 fluid ounces of a 5% (w/v) solution?
A. 91 grains
B. 96 grains
C. 48 grains
D. 100 grains
E. 24 grains

130. An ointment is prepared by incorporating 10 g of a drug into 100 g of white petrolatum. What is the percent w/w of active ingredient?
A. 10.00%
B. 9.10%
C. 0.91%
D. 0.95%
E. None of the above

131. What is the proof strength of a 50% (v/v) solution of alcohol?
A. 25 proof
B. 50 proof
C. 100 proof
D. 75 proof
E. 150 proof

132. Certified dyes may **NOT** be used in the area of
  A. the eye
  B. the scalp
  C. the lips
  D. the nose
  E. all of the above

133. The principal use of magnesium stearate in pharmaceutics is as a (an)
  A. lubricant
  B. antacid
  C. source of Mg ion
  D. disintegrator
  E. binder

134. A synonym for vitamin C is
  A. riboflavin
  B. tocopherol
  C. ascorbic acid
  D. cyanocobalamin
  E. thiamine

135. Activated charcoal is used in some antidotes because of which of its properties?
  A. Neutralizing
  B. Emetic
  C. Absorptive
  D. Adsorptive
  E. Stabilizing

136. What is the pH of a solution that has a hydrogen ion concentration of 1×10^{-8}?
  A. 8.0
  B. 6.0
  C. 1.8
  D. 1.6
  E. None of the above

137. The major use of titanium dioxide in pharmacy is in
  A. sunscreens
  B. antacid tablets

    C. capsules as a diluent
    D. effervescent salts
    E. emulsions

138. Which of the following is used as a hemostatic agent?
    A. Heparin
    B. Oxycel
    C. Coumadins
    D. Indanediones
    E. None of the above

139. Another name for extended insulin zinc suspension is
    A. NPH
    B. Lente
    C. Ultralente
    D. Regular
    E. None of the above

140. The Latin *oculus sinister* means
    A. right eye
    B. left eye
    C. both ears
    D. both eyes
    E. right ear

141. The recommended method of mixing insulins is to
    A. shake vigorously
    B. mix gently by rolling between palms of hands
    C. add simultaneously to container
    D. add lente insulin first then regular insulin
    E. none of the above

142. Membrane filters with 0.22-micron pores can remove which of the following when used to filter solutions?
    A. bacteria
    B. pyrogens
    C. viruses
    D. fungi
    E. A and D

143. Which of the following is **NOT** used as a vehicle for injections?
- **A.** Peanut oil
- **B.** Cottonseed oil
- **C.** Corn oil
- **D.** Theobroma oil
- **E.** Sesame oil

144. Which preservative has recently been removed from several vaccine products to decrease the potential of toxicity events in children?
- **A.** benzyl alcohol
- **B.** sodium bicarbonate
- **C.** thimerosal
- **D.** peanut oil
- **E.** methylparaben

145. Two formulations of different active ingredients that have been judged to produce similar effects are called
- **I.** generic equivalence
- **II.** therapeutic equivalence
- **III.** pharmaceutical equivalence

- **A.** I only
- **B.** III only
- **C.** I and II only
- **D.** II and III only
- **E.** I, II, and III

146. Drugs subject to a significant first-pass effect following oral administration include
- **I.** Propranolol
- **II.** Nifedipine
- **III.** Nitroglycerin

- **A.** I only
- **B.** III only
- **C.** I and II only
- **D.** II and III only
- **E.** I, II, and III

147. Which of the following factors is (are) important in the delivery of drug to the intended site of absorption with a metered dose inhaler?

  I. Particle size and shape
  II. Physiochemical properties of the active ingredient
  III. Use of an oral adaptor

  A. I only
  B. III only
  C. I and II only
  D. II and III only
  E. I, II, and III

148. Which of the following is a true statement regarding transdermal delivery systems?

  A. Products from different manufacturers require identical amounts of active ingredient to yield equivalent responses
  B. Skin thickness is not a factor in drug absorption
  C. The transdermal unit should always be placed at the same site
  D. The transdermal unit contains more drug than is intended for delivery into the body over the prescribed period of use
  E. The transdermal unit may remain attached to the skin after the labeled delivery period because drug absorption ceases

149. Which of the following orders contain the basic components needed for a standard total parenteral nutrition solution?

  A. Dextrose 7.5%, amino acids 4.25%, electrolytes
  B. Dextrose 10%, albumin 4%, multivitamin concentrate 10 mL
  C. Amino acids 15%, insulin 5 units/L, electrolytes
  D. Dextrose 2.5%, fat emulsion 30%, electrolytes
  E. Dextrose 5%, amino acids 30%, fat emulsion 20%

150. The most commonly used method to sterilize talc powder for the treatment of pleural effusions is
   A. gas sterilization
   B. irradiation
   C. low level heat
   D. moist heat
   E. dry heat

Pharmaceutics/ Pharmacokinetics

Answers and Discussion

1. **(C)** Tweens favor o/w emulsions because of high HLB.

2. **(E)** All of the factors affect drug distribution.

3. **(C)** All other orders are dependent on concentration of one or more substances present.

4. **(C)** Spans merely contain fewer oxyethylene groups than tweens.

5. **(A)** Oral doses are metabolized by the liver before reaching systemic circulation.

6. **(E)** Stability and solubility properties may be changed.

7. **(E)** Drugs will be changed or eliminated before diffusion is attained.

8. **(C)** The term rem is a measure of exposure to radioactivity.

9. **(B)** pH is the negative log of the hydrogen ion concentration (or hydronium ion concentration).

10. **(E)** Muscle tissue is the only one of the three types of tissue that seldom stores drugs.

11. (B) Hydrolysis of penicillin G is rapid.

12. (D) Ten percent sulfur paste or ointment is used as an alternative treatment for *Sarcoptes scabiei*. Sulfur is also used as an active keratolytic. At full strength, it is used alone or in combination with other keratolytics, such as salicylic acid. If a patient's skin demonstrates intolerance to sulfur, the concentration should be reduced.

13. (C) If the solutions are not diluted, a false-negative result is common.

14. (C) Vinblastine and vincristine are the drugs obtained from vinca rosea.

15. (A) The drug must be highly un-ionized to penetrate the blood–brain barrier; this process is quite slow in general.

16. (E) Niacin may cause GI upset.

17. (E) Daily dosing is necessary to maintain therapeutic level.

18. (C) The half-life is equal to $0.693/k$ in first-order kinetics.

19. (D) $25 \times 74.6/1000 = 1.86$ g.

20. (D) The sodium present in sodium penicillin G must be included in the sodium count.

21. (D) 87 g/xg $= 1$ Eq/500 cc per 0.01 Eq/500 cc; $x = 0.87$.

22. (C) $74.6 \times 0.05 = 3.73$.

23. (E) The volume of distribution is the proportionality constant between amount of drug in the body and plasma concentration. Immediately after administration of a drug by IV bolus, the amount of drug in the body equals the intravenous dose divided by the volume of distribution.

$$\text{Plasma concentration at time 0 } (C_0) = \frac{\text{IV dose}}{\text{volume of distribution}}$$

24. **(B)** Most drugs are weak acids or weak bases.

25. **(B)** Hydrolysis occurs to some degree with many drugs.

26. **(C)** The equations are named after the scientists who developed them.

27. **(B)** This ion product is obtained by adding the pH and pOH.

28. **(A)** Oxidation pathways are less common in vivo.

29. **(C)** Trough concentrations are indicative of drug accumulation. To decrease only the trough level and maintain peak concentrations, lengthening the dosing interval is the method of choice.

30. **(C)** 0.5 mg/x mg = 2.2 lb/44 lb; x = 100 mg (0.01 g). The patient's age is not relevant.

31. **(D)** Volume = weight/density. Thus,
volume = 30 g/1.8 g/mL = 16.67 mL

32. **(A)** Weight = density × volume. Thus,
weight = 1.18 g/mL × 25 mL = 29.500 g

33. **(A)** For most drugs, biotransformation results in conversion to a more polar compound, which is more easily cleared by the kidney.

34. **(D)** The optimal loading dose is easily estimated by use of the following formula:

$$\text{Loading dose} = \text{desired plasma concentration} \times \text{volume of distribution}$$

35. **(B)** 15.4 grains = 1 gram. Thus,
60 grams × 15.4 grains/gram = 924 grains.

36. **(B)** It is a classic type of first-order reaction.

37. **(C)** It is a measure of oil and water balance in emulsions.

38. (B) Alpha particles and helium atoms have the same mass.

39. (D) Both adjustment of dosage interval and dosage size reduction are acceptable methods for decreasing drug accumulation in patients with renal failure. The two methods may be used in combination, depending on the dosage forms available, the therapeutic range, and convenience.

40. (C) Corn or potato starch is used.

41. (D) These fluorinated hydrocarbons are used as propellants in aerosols.

42. (D) The liver and kidneys commonly become less functional in the elderly.

43. (B) Assume 16 oz/pint, and 30 mL/oz. Thus,

$$2 \text{ pt} \times 16 \text{ oz/pt} = 32 \text{ oz}$$

$$(32 \text{ oz} \times 30 \text{ mL/oz}) + (3 \text{ oz} \times 30 \text{ mL/oz}) = 960 \text{ mL} + 90 \text{ mL}$$

$$= 1050 \text{ mL}$$

44. (E) Less than 3.5 kg hardness tablets cause fragmentation during shipping.

45. (A) Protamine sulfate is the primary antidote.

46. (B) 96 mg/0.6 mg/dose =160 doses

47. (B) Dextrans are inert and soluble, so they cause no problems.

48. (A) The term *ppm* is typically used in expressing concentrations of very dilute preparations and is defined as "parts per million."

49. (C) These are good manufacturing practices.

50. (D) At this point acid/base is 1.0. The log of 1 is 0; therefore, pH = pka.

51. **(D)** The Bronsted–Lowry theory is the proton donor–acceptor theory of acids and bases.

52. **(E)** Salicylic acid is used in topicals to cause sloughing of skin.

53. **(A)** Pyridoxine is the synonym for B_6.

54. **(C)** $473 \text{ g} \times 8 \times 1.25 = 4730.0 \text{ g}$

55. **(D)** Vitamin K is necessary for formation of prothrombin.

56. **(D)** Cobalt is an element in the chemical structure.

57. **(C)** Carbowax is a trade name used for this group.

58. **(C)** $°F = 9/5 \, (-12°C) + 32 = 10.4°F$

59. **(A)** One tablespoon is about one-half ounce, or 15 mL.

60. **(E)** More than 10,000 parts of solvent per one part of solute is considered practically insoluble or insoluble.

61. **(D)** 190 proof is 95% alcohol.

$$70/95 = x/500$$

$$x = 368 \text{ cc}$$

62. **(B)** Dose forms of aerosols are covered by the Federal Hazardous Substance Labeling Act because they are in pressurized containers, which could explode.

63. **(C)** Magnesium controls convulsions by locking neuromuscular response.

64. **(A)** Barium sulfate creates an opaque medium for x-ray.

65. **(C)** The American Council on Pharmaceutical Education accredits all schools.

66. **(A)** If creaming or reversible precipitation occurs, the emulsion can be reestablished. Change of phase does not always result in precipitation.

67. (E) Pyrogens can commonly cause all of the symptoms listed.

68. (B) In this process, water is sublimed from a frozen product. The other answers represent different processes.

69. (E) Lubricants such as talc or stearates facilitate all three functions.

70. (C) Tablets comprise about 75% of all solid dosage forms, followed by hard capsules (23%), and soft elastic capsules (2%).

71. (D) Veegum is a synthetic hydrophilic thickening agent.

72. (A) Sorbitol renders the shells elastic. It can also be used as a thickener or emulsifier, but only in liquid dose forms.

73. (D) Capsules for human use are available in sizes from 000 (largest) to 5 (smallest). Size 0000 would be too large to swallow.

74. (E) The three applications listed are the main uses of ointment: to soften, to protect, and to serve as a semisolid carrier.

75. (C) A humectant such as glycerin helps to retain moisture and prevent drying due to evaporation.

76. (D) The Noyes–Whitney equation is used to determine dissolution rate and does not describe any other biopharmaceutical functions.

77. (E) Starch in the form of a paste can serve as a binder. It also exhibits glidant properties and can help with disintegration when it comes in contact with body fluids.

78. (E) All are characteristics of flocculated particles in a suspension. The rate of sedimentation is high, because particles settles as a floc (a collection of particles). Although a sediment is formed rapidly, it is loosely packed and possess a scaffold-like structure. Because the particles do not bond tightly, caking does not occur. The suspension may not appear uniform due to rapid sedimentation.

79. **(D)** Gums are effective only as binders. They increase hardness and tend to impede lubrication or flow.

80. **(E)** All three statements are true because these tablets must dissolve in the mouth readily and they bypass GI tract absorption.

81. **(D)** Vanishing creams are emulsion bases of the o/w type and contain a high percentage of water.

82. **(A)** Although syrup NF has a high enough concentration of sucrose to retard bacterial growth, it is not a saturated solution. This ensures good stability.

83. **(C)** Only hydrochloric acid is a strong acid; it donates protons readily. Concentration is not the criterion used.

84. **(B)** Temperature increase has a marked effect on reaction rate, whereas the other choices have a negative effect, no effect, or only cause slight increases.

85. **(D)** Increase of surface area and reduction of particle size promote faster dissolution, whereas aggregation impedes dissolution.

86. **(C)** Units for renal clearance involve the volume of drug-containing plasma removed by the kidney per unit of time, and not the concentration of drug.

87. **(D)** GMP regulations are good manufacturing practices and are administered by the Food and Drug Administration.

88. **(A)** Ethylene glycol may oxidize to form oxalic acid, which is corrosive and quite toxic.

89. **(B)** Glucose is a simple sugar that cannot be hydrolized, but it is water soluble.

90. **(C)**   Purified water USP can be used in oral preparations, but it may contain pyrogens and is not suitable for parenterals.

91. **(B)**   Ferritin is a micelle of ferric hydroxyphosphate surrounded by protein units.

92. **(D)**   Pyridoxine is vitamin B_6. The rest are other vitamins in the B complex.

93. **(A)**   HLB is an acronym for hydrophile–lipophile balance, and is used to classify surfactants as emulsifiers. The other answers deal with terms used in tabletting or suspensions.

94. **(D)**   Chlorobutanol suffers from all of the disadvantages listed and, in addition, is very slow acting.

95. **(A)**   A solution has an osmolal concentration of one when it contains 1 osmol of solute/kg of water

96. **(B)**   It takes 2 hours to penetrate the horny layer of the skin and provide maximum protection.

97. **(E)**   Zinc salts enhance the fungistatic action, but also increase sensitivity.

98. **(A)**   Vitamins A, D, E, and K are fat soluble. The others are water soluble.

99. **(E)**   The most effective saline laxatives are magnesium and sulfate ions, which are dibasic and relatively nonabsorbable.

100. **(C)**   Bismuth subsalicylate is an effective absorbent that can absorb toxins, bacteria, and fluids; it has no inherent antimicrobial activity.

101. **(A)**   Sublimation is a transformation of solid to vapor without going through the liquid state.

102. **(D)**   This is a quarternary ammonium compound, which is cationic. The others are anionic emulsifiers.

103. (E) Mineral oil acts only by lubricating the intestinal tract. It has very mild or secondary properties of fecal softening.

104. (B) This substance is impervious to gastric juices and dissolves in intestinal fluids. It has no other pharmaceutical use.

105. (B) It melts at about 37°C (body temperature) and releases the drug.

106. (D) Moist heat is the method of choice because of its dependability, effectiveness, and low cost. The other methods are used when moist heat cannot be used.

107. (E) All of these properties should be achieved, in addition to stability and clarity.

108. (B) The concentrations must be expressed in moles to account for differences in molecular weight, which affects ionization.

109. (C) If the salt:acid concentration is 1:1, the salt:acid term is equal to the log of 1, which is 0, and this term is dropped. Therefore, the pH is equal to the pKa.

110. (B) The buffer equation was named for the two men who developed it.

111. (D) An ampholyte is a substance capable of functioning as both an acid and a base. All except NaH_2PO_4 can function only as either an acid or a base.

112. (D) Soda lime is used to absorb carbon dioxide in anesthesia machines, oxygen therapy, and metabolic tests only.

113. (E) Pumice is useful as an abrasive in cleansing agents or dentifrices, and as a filtering agent.

114. (C) The original Food and Drug Act of 1906 and the 1938 Food, Drug, and Cosmetic Act did not require proof of efficacy. It was not until 1962 that the Kefauver–Harris amendment required proof of efficacy.

115. (D) *Bleeding* is used to describe separation of liquid ingredients from ointment bases only.

116. (D) Although regulations were first issued in 1963, they did not become official until 1979, after several revisions.

117. (A) The Limulus test is an in vitro test for pyrogens and is more rapid, sensitive, and simple than the rabbit test.

118. (A) Excessive infusion of hypotonic solutions may cause hemolysis and water intoxication. Clinical results included convulsions with edema, including pulmonary edema.

119. (E) Excessive infusions of hypertonic dextrose solutions (rich in dextrose) may cause loss of electrolytes, hyperglycemia, intracellular dehydration, glycosuria, and osmotic diuresis. Clinical effects may include dehydration and coma.

120. (E) Rectal temperatures typically run about 1° higher than oral. In establishing normal temperature, it is common to take temperatures several times during the day to establish an average.

121. (B) This Latin term is translated as "each eye" or "both eyes."

122. (E) Liquid forms are usually less stable and may have an objectionable taste. The necessity to measure teaspoons makes dosage less predictable and accurate.

123. (C) Oral contraceptives are exempt because of their unique and useful design. Nitroglycerin is exempt because of the need for direct and immediate access. Oral analgesics are not exempt unless requested by the physician or patient.

124. (A) The Latin *post cibos* can be translated to mean "after meals."

125. (D) Compressed gases possess little expansion power and tend to produce wet sprays or foaming. They are usually inert and have no other adverse effect.

126. (C) Although it is related to other corticosteroids, it is not possible for the liver enzymes to convert to anything other than prednisolone.

127. (E) All three statements are true.

128. (B) 1 kg = 2.2 lb. By proportion:

$$\frac{5 \text{ mg}}{x \text{ mg}} = \frac{2.2 \text{ lb}}{110 \text{ lb}}$$

$$x = 250 \text{ mg}$$

129. (A) 1 oz/4 oz = 455/x gr; 1820 gr × 0.05 = 91 gr

130. (C) 10 g/x = 110/100; x = 9.1%

131. (C) The proof strength of alcohol is double the v/v percentage strength

132. (A) Some certified dyes may be used in all areas; however, no category of dye may be applied to the area of the eye because of the potential for damage.

133. (A) Magnesium stearate is a free-flowing insoluble compound used as a lubricant in granulations or powder mixtures. It has no other use.

134. (C) The other names are synonyms for other vitamins.

135. (D) Activated charcoal is capable of adsorbing a number of toxins because of its high specific surface.

136. (A) The log of 1 is 0. The log of 10^{-8} is 8, so the pH of 0 + 8 = 8.

137. (A) Titanium dioxide in proper concentration can completely block the burning rays of the sun.

138. (B) Oxicel is an absorbable gelatin sponge that promotes clotting. The other drugs tend to prevent clotting.

139. (C) Ultralente insulin contains large crystals of insulin with a high zinc content that are collected and resuspended in a sodium acetate/sodium chloride solution.

140. (B) The Latin *oculus sinister* means left eye.

141. (B) Vigorous shaking may break protein structures.

142. (E) Due to their larger size, bacteria and fungi can be removed by using a 0.22-micron filter. Viruses are too small and will pass through the filter. Pyrogens are most commonly destroyed by heat.

143. (D) Theobroma oil is a semisolid at room temperature and is used as a suppository base.

144. (C) A review conducted by the FDA concluded that the use of thimerosal as a preservative in vaccines might result in the intake of mercury during the first 6 months of life that exceeds EPA recommendations. Today all vaccines in the recommended childhood immunization schedule that are for use in the U.S. market contain no thimerosal or only trace amounts (<0.0002%). Influenza (flu) vaccines and tetanus and diphtheria vaccines (Td and DT) are not available without thimerosal. Information on thimerosal content in manufactured U.S. licensed vaccines can be found at <www.fda.gov/cber/vaccine/thimcnt.htm>.

145. (B) The terms *generic equivalent* and *pharmaceutical equivalent* refer to medications identical in active ingredient, strength, and dosage form.

146. (E) Propranolol, nifedipine, and nitroglycerin are all subject to extensive metabolism by the liver prior to the drug reaching the systemic circulation.

147. (E) Particle size and shape, solubility of active ingredient in pulmonary fluids, and configuration of the oral adaptor to reduce oropharyngeal deposition of aerosol are all important factors in aerosol delivery of the drug.

148. (D)   Transdermal units contain much greater quantities of active ingredient than is delivered over the intended period of use. The drug delivery rate decreases as the concentration in the unit falls but it does not necessarily cease at the end of the prescribed delivery period.

149. (A)   Essential components in parenteral nutrition solutions are amino acids, dextrose, electrolytes, vitamins, and trace elements. Generally, peripheral solutions contain 5% to 7.5% dextrose and 3% to 5% amino acids. A dextrose concentration of 10% or greater should be infused through a central venous line.

150. (A)   Gas sterilization is one of the more common methods used to sterilize powders, particularly talc.

2

Pharmacology

DIRECTIONS (Questions 1–215): Each of the questions or incomplete statements below is followed by five suggested answers or completions. Select the **one answer** that is best in each case.

1. Etanercept is used mainly to treat
   A. gout
   B. arthritis
   C. diabetes
   D. carcinomas
   E. high blood pressure

2. Dosage of anticonvulsants is adjusted
   A. when seizures occur frequently
   B. every 2 weeks
   C. every 2 years
   D. only when side effects are seen
   E. seasonally

3. Which of the following symptoms is **NOT** present in digitalis intoxication?
   A. AV block
   B. Ventricular tachycardia
   C. Vomiting
   D. Vagal arrest of the heart
   E. Visual disturbances

4. Sulfonamides are excreted free and combined as
   A. the acetyl derivative
   B. the amino derivative
   C. the sulfate derivative
   D. the glycine conjugate
   E. none of the above

5. Which of the following agents is associated with tinnitus as a result of toxicity?
   A. salicylate
   B. phenytoin
   C. propranolol
   D. acetaminophen
   E. cyclobenzaprine

6. Parkinsonism is probably due to
   A. too little dopamine in the brain
   B. too little levodopa in the brain
   C. too little acetylcholine in the brain
   D. too much levodopa in the brain
   E. too much dopamine in the brain

7. The greatest threat from morphine poisoning is
   A. renal shutdown
   B. paralysis of spinal cord
   C. respiratory depression
   D. cardiovascular collapse
   E. none of the above

8. A specific narcotic antagonist is
   A. meperidine
   B. polybrene
   C. nalorphine
   D. universal antidote
   E. meprobamate

9. Which of the following is used to curtail chronic uric acid stone formation?
   A. Allopurinol
   B. Trimethoprim
   C. Methenamine
   D. Ethacrynic acid
   E. Furosemide

10. Which of the following is used to lower blood lipid levels?
    A. Trimethadione
    B. Colesevelam
    C. Flucytosine
    D. Coumarin
    E. Propranolol

11. Therapeutically, vitamin B_1 has been used most successfully in the treatment of
    A. microcytic anemia
    B. pellagra
    C. scurvy
    D. beriberi
    E. macrocytic anemia

12. Capecitabine is used to treat
    A. hypertension
    B. muscular injuries
    C. ulcers
    D. breast cancer
    E. congestive heart failure

13. Magnesium ion is necessary in
    A. stimulating enzyme systems
    B. muscular contraction
    C. nerve conduction
    D. all of the above
    E. none of the above

14. A class of plant alkaloids widely used to treat migraine is
    A. vinca alkaloids
    B. digitalis glycosides
    C. stramonium alkaloids

    D. ergot alkaloids
    E. belladonna alkaloids

15. Complications of enteral tube feedings include
    A. aspiration pneumonia
    B. diarrhea
    C. hyperglycemia
    D. fluid and electrolyte disturbances
    E. all of the above

16. Which of the following drugs is used to "rescue" patients who have received high-dose methotrexate?
    A. Allopurinol
    B. Leucovorin
    C. Methyldopa
    D. Naloxone
    E. Isoflurane

17. Cyclosporine is used for
    A. allergies
    B. angina
    C. prevention of transplant rejection
    D. steroid deficiency
    E. treating lead poisoning

18. Pantoprazole is used primarily to treat
    A. gastric hyperacidity
    B. hypertension
    C. cardiac insufficiency
    D. gout
    E. migraine headache

19. Citalopram is a (an)
    A. diuretic
    B. cardiotonic
    C. antidepressant
    D. anti-inflammatory
    E. anthelmintic

20. Daunorubicin and doxorubicin have been commonly associated with
   A. ulcers
   B. cardiac toxicity
   C. colitis
   D. gout
   E. hepatotoxicity

21. In which of the following dosage forms is nicotine available when used as a smoking deterrent?
   A. transdermal
   B. nasal spray
   C. gum
   D. A and C
   E. A, B, and C

22. Triamcinolone differs from most glucocorticoids because it does **NOT**
   A. cause depression
   B. cause water retention
   C. affect blood sugar
   D. increase susceptibility to infection
   E. increase appetite

23. Which of the following statements about propylthiouracil is **FALSE**?
   A. It is used for the treatment of hyperthyroidism
   B. It inhibits the synthesis of thyroid hormones
   C. It diminishes peripheral deiodination of T_4 to T_3
   D. It inhibits iodide oxidation
   E. It interferes with the effectiveness of exogenously administered thyroid hormones

24. Folic acid administration has been recommended during pregnancy to prevent which of the following congenital problems?
   A. spina bifida
   B. cystic fibrosis
   C. patent ductus arteriosus
   D. limb deformations
   E. cleft palate

25. Which of the following chemotherapy agents requires a special restricted distribution program due to severe teratogenetic effects?
    A. Vincristine
    B. Cisplatin
    C. 5-fluoruracil
    D. Thalidomide
    E. Cyclophosphamide

26. Which of the following agents is commonly administered with isoniazid to prevent or relieve the symptoms of peripheral neuritis?
    A. Niacin
    B. Pyridoxine
    C. Cyanocobalamin
    D. Ascorbic acid
    E. Acetaminophen

27. An advantage of amoxicillin over ampicillin is that it
    A. is more acid stable
    B. is not destroyed by penicillinase
    C. has a broader spectrum
    D. does not cause allergies
    E. has a longer shelf life

28. Balsalazide is used to treat
    A. hypertension
    B. coronary occlusions
    C. rheumatoid arthritis
    D. diabetes
    E. none of the above

29. Arsenic trioxide was approved by the FDA in 2000 to treat which of the following diseases?
    A. Leukemia
    B. Muscle spasms
    C. Parkinson's disease
    D. Neuralgias
    E. Colon cancer

30. Primidone, used in the treatment of generalized tonic-clonic seizures, is metabolized to
  A. phenytoin
  B. phenobarbital
  C. metformin
  D. carbamazepine
  E. none of the above

31. Vincristine has been commonly associated with which of the following adverse events?
  A. Neurotoxicity
  B. Gout
  C. Duodenal ulcers
  D. Blood clotting
  E. None of the above

32. Dolasetron, a 5-HT$_3$ antagonist is a (an)
  A. β-adrenergic blocker
  B. antiemetic
  C. glucocorticoid
  D. local anesthetic
  E. sunscreen

33. Botulinum toxin is FDA approved to treat
  A. blepharospams
  B. cervical dystonias
  C. facial wrinkles
  D. A and B
  E. A, B, and C

34. Minocycline hydrochloride is a member of which class of anti-infectives?
  A. Cephalosporin
  B. Penicillin
  C. Aminoglycoside
  D. Tetracycline
  E. Sulfonamide

35. Cholestyramine resin has the prevalent side effect of
  A. blocking absorption of some vitamins
  B. raising cholesterol levels

    C. causing intoxication
    D. increasing sensitivity to UV light
    E. all of the above

36. All of the following are diuretics **EXCEPT**
    A. aminophylline
    B. glyburide
    C. spironolactone
    D. bumetamide
    E. chlorthalidone

37. Which of the following is (are) true for tetracyclines?
    I. They may cause yellowing of the teeth in adolescents
    II. They are bacteriostatic
    III. They exhibit a broad spectrum of activity

    A. I only
    B. III only
    C. I and II only
    D. II and III only
    E. I, II, and III

38. Gatifloxacin is a member of which class of anti-infectives?
    A. Cephalosporin
    B. Penicillin
    C. Aminoglycoside
    D. Tetracycline
    E. Fluoroquinolones

39. Infliximab is used to treat
    A. hay fever
    B. vertigo
    C. drug allergies
    D. Crohn's disease
    E. drowsiness

40. Lorazepam produces which of the following action(s)?
    A. Sedation
    B. Loss of memory
    C. Reduction of anxiety
    D. All of the above
    E. None of the above

41. Celecoxib is used as a (an)
   A. antimalarial
   B. cardiotonic
   C. antihistaminic
   D. antacid
   E. analgesic

42. Timolide combines the action of a nonselective beta blocking agent and a (an)
   A. diuretic
   B. cardiotonic
   C. selective beta blocker
   D. anti-inflammatory agent
   E. vasoconstrictor

43. Which of the following drugs has been associated with Reye's syndrome in children?
   A. Aspirin
   B. Acetaminophen
   C. Ibuprofen
   D. Naproxen
   E. Phenobarbital

44. Ultra–short-acting barbiturates are used primarily as
   A. sedatives
   B. hypnotics
   C. antispasmodic agents
   D. anti-parkinsonian agents
   E. preanesthetic agents

45. Norethindrone is a drug commonly used in
   A. mixed estrogens
   B. oral contraceptives
   C. treating carcinomas
   D. diagnostic testing
   E. abortifacients

46. Some anticonvulsants (e.g., carbamazepine, phenytoin, gabapentin) are FDA approved to treat seizures but have also been effective in the treatment of
   A. parkinsonism
   B. neuralgias or neuropathies

C. colitis
D. nausea
E. all of the above

47. Efavirenz is classified as a (an)
A. muscle relaxant
B. sedative–hypnotic
C. tranquilizer
D. analgesic
E. antiviral

48. Lepirudin is used mainly to treat
A. gastritis
B. minor anxiety states
C. heparin-induced thrombocytopenia
D. severe pain
E. nausea

49. Histamine is found in the human body in
A. the granules of mast cells in blood
B. the mucosal layer of the GI tract
C. the hypothalamus
D. A and B
E. A, B, and C

50. Orlistat is used as a (an)
A. narcotic antagonist
B. narcotic analgesic
C. weight loss agent
D. antiepileptic
E. anesthetic

51. Which of the following is **NOT** a side effect of codeine?
A. Miosis
B. Nausea
C. Diarrhea
D. Respiratory depression
E. Addiction

52. Antipsychotics usually act on the
  A. cerebrum
  B. cerebellum
  C. lower brain areas
  D. brain and spinal cord
  E. nerve endings

53. Lidocaine is used as a local anesthetic or as a (an)
  A. general anesthetic
  B. antipruritic
  C. preanesthetic
  D. antiarrhythmic
  E. analgesic

54. Cocaine has a long duration of local anesthetic action because it is
  A. more stable than most local anesthetics
  B. readily absorbed
  C. not biotransformed
  D. a vasoconstrictor
  E. none of the above

55. All of the following are natural estrogens or congeners **EXCEPT**
  A. estradiol
  B. diethylstilbestrol
  C. estrone
  D. ethinyl estradiol
  E. estropipate

56. Which of the following is used to treat hyperthyroidism?
  A. Liotrix
  B. Thyroglobulin
  C. Liothyronine
  D. Propylthiouracil
  E. Etidronate

57. Carbidopa is used to
  A. treat Parkinson's disease
  B. treat hypertension
  C. potentiate levodopa

D. treat depression

E. treat Gehrig's disease

58. Hyoscyamine has the same action as atropine but is

A. twice as potent

B. three times more potent

C. ten times more potent

D. half as potent

E. one-fourth as potent

59. Gemtuzumab is used primarily as a (an)

A. cardiotonic

B. antidepressant

C. diuretic

D. antineoplastic

E. sedative

60. The principal toxic effect of heparin is

A. hemorrhage

B. bronchospasm

C. chills

D. fever

E. hair loss

61. Tenecteplase is used primarily to reduce mortality associated with which of the following clinical problems?

A. Diabetes

B. Myocardial infarction

C. Hemorrhage

D. Prostate cancer

E. None of the above

62. Albuterol is usually administered by which route?

A. IV

B. IM

C. Nasal

D. Rectal

E. Oral

63. Nateglinide is used most commonly to treat
   A. AIDS
   B. genital herpes
   C. diabetes
   D. CMV retinitis
   E. influenza

64. Barbiturates, in general, are particularly noted for
   A. lack of habituation
   B. producing microsomal enzymes in liver
   C. instability
   D. slow absorption
   E. poor oral absorption

65. Meloxicam exerts its action because it is a (an)
   A. nonsteroidal anti-inflammatory
   B. MAO inhibitor
   C. alkaline
   D. calcium channel blocker
   E. acid

66. The principal mechanism of action of penicillins on micro-organisms is
   A. inhibition of cell wall synthesis
   B. destruction of the nucleus
   C. bacteriostatic
   D. causing mutations
   E. lysis

67. Epinephrine is **NOT** given orally because
   A. it is inactivated in the gastric mucosa
   B. local vasoconstriction inhibits absorption
   C. it is rapidly inactivated in circulation
   D. of none of the above
   E. of all of the above

68. Which of the following cardiac glycosides does **NOT** occur naturally?
   A. Digoxin
   B. Ouabain
   C. Digitoxin

D. Amrinone
E. Nitroglycerin

69. Oxcarbazepine is used to treat
    A. partial seizures
    B. Hodgkin's disease
    C. angina pectoris
    D. breast cancer
    E. depression

70. Which of the following is classified as a cholinergic antagonist?
    A. Acetylcholine
    B. Neostigmine
    C. Atropine
    D. Bethanecol
    E. Methacholine

71. The action of heparin is terminated by
    A. coumarin
    B. indanediones
    C. insulins
    D. sulfonamides
    E. protamine sulfate

72. Nitroglycerin has a relatively short half-life due to
    A. its volatility
    B. its chemical instability
    C. its poor absorption
    D. first-pass metabolism
    E. all of the above

73. Various opiates may be used as all of the following **EXCEPT**
    A. analgesics
    B. anti-inflammatories
    C. antidiarrheals
    D. aids to anesthesia
    E. antitussives

74. Trihexylphenidyl is used to treat
    A. parkinsonism
    B. angina
    C. xerostomia
    D. glaucoma
    E. muscle spasms

75. The prevalent mechanism of action of antihistaminics is that they
    A. prevent formation of histamine
    B. speed up elimination of histamine
    C. destroy histamine
    D. competitively inhibit histamine
    E. speed up biotransformation of histamine

76. Isotretinoin is commonly used to treat
    A. lice infestations
    B. fungal infestations
    C. ringworm
    D. burns
    E. acne

77. Endorphins play a significant role in
    A. pain perception
    B. absorption
    C. diuresis
    D. hypertension
    E. glaucoma

78. The most effective substance in treating acute attacks of gout is
    A. allopurinol
    B. probenecid
    C. aspirin
    D. para-aminobenzoic acid
    E. colchicine

79. Nystatin is used to treat
    A. *Trichomonas* infestations
    B. *Staphylococcus aureus* infections
    C. candidiasis

    D. *Escherichia coli* infections
    E. rickettsial infections

80. Which of the following NSAIDs is available in a parenteral form?
    A. ibuprofen
    B. ketorolac
    C. tolmetin
    D. piroxicam
    E. none of the above

81. Muscle relaxants are seldom used for more than 2 to 3 weeks because
    A. of toxicity
    B. of instability
    C. of short duration of need
    D. of tolerance being developed
    E. they are used longer commonly

82. Linezolid is used against infections caused by antibiotic-resistant
    A. gram-positive cocci
    B. gram-negative bacilli
    C. HIV virus
    D. gram-positive bacilli
    E. none of the above

83. Nateglinide stimulates the release of
    A. insulin
    B. epinephrine
    C. glucose
    D. glucagon
    E. norepinephrine

84. Mifeprostone is a receptor antagonist of which hormone?
    A. Estrogen
    B. Thyroid
    C. Insulin
    D. Cortisol
    E. Progesterone

85. Rivastigmine has the primary action of inhibiting
   A. acetyl cholinesterase
   B. epinephrine
   C. gastric acid
   D. calcium influx
   E. histamine release

86. Which of the following are low-molecular-weight heparins?
   A. Tinzaparin
   B. Enoxaparin
   C. Dalteparin
   D. B and C
   E. A, B, and C

87. Ocular timolol is used primarily in
   A. glaucoma
   B. pink eye
   C. conjunctivitis
   D. eye infections
   E. eye cleansers

88. Sucralfate is used for short-term therapy of
   A. ulcers
   B. hypertension
   C. carcinomas
   D. calcium depletion
   E. dental caries

89. Lorazepam is classified as a
   A. loop diuretic
   B. MAO inhibitor
   C. thiazide diuretic
   D. dibenzazepine
   E. polycyclic amine

90. Probantheline is contraindicated in patients with
   A. glaucoma
   B. myasthenia gravis
   C. obstructive disease of GI tract
   D. ulcerative colitis
   E. all of the above

91. Antiepileptics as a group are noted for developing or causing
    A. rashes
    B. atrial tachycardias
    C. tolerance
    D. spasms
    E. headache

92. Selenium sulfide is used
    A. orally
    B. topically
    C. by injection
    D. by none of the above
    E. by all of the above

93. Zonisamide is considered a broad-spectrum
    A. antibiotic
    B. anticonvulsant
    C. antiviral
    D. NSAID
    E. antihistamine

94. Which of the following is **NOT** a stimulant laxative?
    A. Cascara sagrada
    B. Senna
    C. Castor oil
    D. Bisacodyl
    E. Docusate

95. Which of the following actions is **NOT** seen with sympathomimetics?
    A. Pupil constriction
    B. Increased heart rate
    C. Sweat gland stimulation
    D. Bronchiole dilation
    E. Systemic blood vessel constriction

96. Baclofen is used primarily as a (an)
    A. sympathomimetic
    B. antianxiety agent
    C. muscle relaxant
    D. antispasmodic
    E. tranquilizer

97. Beta-interferon is used to treat
  A. adult-onset diabetes
  B. hypertension
  C. cardiac insufficiency
  D. multiple sclerosis
  E. ulcers

98. A prevalent side effect of propylthiouracil is
  A. hearing loss
  B. visual impairment
  C. acidosis
  D. leukopenia
  E. muscular spasm

99. Candesartan is used as a (an)
  A. diuretic
  B. antihypertensive
  C. hypnotic
  D. sedative
  E. antidepressant

100. The pharmacologic actions of sulindac include
  I. anti-inflammatory properties
  II. analgesic properties
  III. antipyretic properties

  A. I only
  B. II only
  C. I and II only
  D. I and III only
  E. I, II, and III

101. Mirtazapine is used to treat symptoms of
  A. depression
  B. parkinsonism
  C. gout
  D. petit mal epilepsy
  E. none of the above

102. Ofloxacin is classified as a (an)
  A. antifungal
  B. antiviral

C. broad-spectrum antibiotic
D. narrow-spectrum antibiotic
E. antirickettsial

103. Zidovudine may commonly cause which of the following as a side effect?
A. Vasoconstriction
B. Dryness of the mouth
C. Hyperactivity
D. Anemia
E. Anuria

104. Mupirocin ointment is used topically to treat
A. conjunctivitis
B. all types of eye infections
C. impetigo
D. carcinomas of the skin
E. hemorrhoids

105. Pentoxifylline acts primarily by
A. dissolving cholesterol
B. decreasing viscosity of the blood
C. increasing biotransformation
D. oxidative mechanisms
E. preventing formation of cholesterol

106. Which of the following is most useful in treating a hypertensive crisis?
A. Sodium nitroprusside
B. Serpasil
C. Chlorothiazide
D. Spironolactone
E. Triamterene

107. Allopurinol differs from most other agents used to treat gouty conditions because it
A. does not decrease uric acid levels
B. prevents formation of uric acid
C. increases elimination of uric acid
D. causes rapid biotransformation of uric acid
E. has analgesic properties

108. Estrogens tend to increase the risk of
  A. endometrial carcinoma
  B. hirsutism
  C. hearing loss
  D. visual problems
  E. pregnancy

109. Which of the following drugs is contraindicated when used with sildenafil?
  A. Fluoroquinolones
  B. Organic nitrates
  C. Penicillins
  D. Calcium channel blockers
  E. None of the above

110. Gentamicin exhibits
  A. significant hepatotoxicity
  B. significant cardiotoxicity
  C. significant dermal toxicity
  D. significant nephrotoxicity
  E. all of the above

111. Risendronate is classified as a (an)
  A. cardiosuppressant
  B. bisphosphonate
  C. diuretic
  D. immunosuppressant
  E. sympathomimetic

112. Carbamazepine is used as an anticonvulsant as well as to treat pain from
  A. kidney infections
  B. burns
  C. muscle injuries
  D. sinus headache
  E. trigeminal neuralgia

113. Methylphenidate is used to treat
  A. fatigue
  B. hyperkinesis disorders
  C. anxiety

    D. depression

    E. obesity

114. Doxorubicin is used to treat

    A. a wide variety of infections

    B. gram-positive infections

    C. gram-negative infections

    D. viral infections

    E. carcinomas

115. A drug that is useful in treating potentially fatal fungal infections is

    A. nystatin

    B. propionic acid

    C. amphotericin B

    D. nystatin

    E. griseofulvin

116. The use of thyroid hormones in the treatment of obesity is

    A. widely accepted

    B. unjustified

    C. acceptable in combination with other drugs

    D. only acceptable if other treatments fail

    E. acceptable if the patient is closely monitored

117. An advantage of dextromethorphan over codeine as an antitussive is that it

    A. is twice as effective

    B. is more stable

    C. has no side effects

    D. produces very little depression of the CNS

    E. has better analgesic properties

118. Nonselective 2-adrenoreceptor antagonists are used primarily in

    A. peripheral vascular disorders

    B. tachycardia

    C. migraine headache

    D. atherosclerosis

    E. renal insufficiency

119. All of the following statements about propranolol are true **EXCEPT**
  A. the oral route of administration is preferred
  B. propranolol penetrates into the CNS
  C. propranolol is primarily biotransformed in the liver
  D. propranolol causes rashes and sore throat
  E. it is a nonselective alpha antagonist

120. Antimuscarinic drugs are contraindicated in
  A. narrow angle glaucoma
  B. paralytic ilens
  C. pyloric or intestinal obstruction
  D. A and B
  E. A, B, and C

121. Zanamivir and ostelamivir are both FDA approved for
  A. treatment of influenza A infection
  B. treatment of influenza B infection
  C. prophylaxis of influenza infections
  D. A and B
  E. A, B, and C

122. Which of the following drugs is not a proton pump inhibitor?
  A. Pantoprazole
  B. Rabeprazole
  C. Lansoprazole
  D. Sulfisoxazole
  E. Omeprazole

123. A danger of prolonged use of pilocarpine salts as a miotic is
  A. tearing
  B. glaucoma
  C. conjunctivitis
  D. detached retina
  E. lens opacity

124. A serious side effect of furosemide in treating heart patients is that it
  A. interacts with digitalis glycosides
  B. causes arterial blockage
  C. may cause anuria

    D. causes hypertension
    E. may lose its effect

125. All of the following are side effects of progestins **EXCEPT**
    A. weight gain
    B. headache
    C. fatigue
    D. constipation
    E. nausea and vomiting

126. Which of the following drugs require electrocardiographic monitoring prior to initiation of therapy?
    A. Ziprasidone
    B. Arsenic trioxide
    C. Cisapride
    D. A and B
    E. A, B, and C

127. Lamivudine is usually classified as a (an)
    A. H_2 antagonist
    B. ulcer protectant
    C. antiviral
    D. oral antidiabetic
    E. anthelmintic

128. Prolonged usage of sublingual nitrates is likely to cause
    A. ulcers
    B. anuria
    C. rashes
    D. development of tolerance
    E. persistent headache

129. Streptokinase is used to
    A. dissolve blood clots
    B. treat digestive disorders
    C. promote carbohydrate degradation
    D. treat muscle injuries
    E. replace pepsin

130. Gold compounds have been used to treat
    A. worm infestations
    B. ulcers
    C. kidney failure
    D. rheumatoid arthritis
    E. psoriasis

131. Tamoxifen is classified as a (an)
    A. estrogen
    B. antiestrogen
    C. androsterone
    D. testosterone
    E. thyroid hormone

132. Bacitracin is **NOT** usually given parenterally because of its
    A. insolubility
    B. lack of stability
    C. pain at the injection site
    D. lack of potency
    E. nephrotoxicity

133. Beriberi is associated with a deficiency of
    A. vitamin D
    B. thiamine
    C. vitamin C
    D. niacin
    E. riboflavin

134. A drug used to treat delirium tremens is
    A. chlordiazepoxide
    B. haloperidol
    C. disulfiram
    D. methadone
    E. none of the above

135. Cromolyn sodium acts by
    A. destroying histamine
    B. releasing histamine
    C. biotransforming histamine
    D. preventing the release of histamine
    E. none of the above

136. The anti-inflammatory action of aspirin is due to
    A. analgesia
    B. inhibition of clotting
    C. antipyretic effect
    D. degradation of prostaglandins
    E. inhibition of prostaglandin synthesis

137. Castor oil is classified as which type of laxative?
    A. Lubricating
    B. Anthraquinone
    C. Irritant
    D. Stool softening
    E. Bulk producing

138. Penicillamine is most commonly used to treat
    A. parkinsonism
    B. Wilson's disease
    C. neoplasms
    D. Raynaud's disease
    E. gram-positive infections

139. Which of the following drugs was withdrawn from the U.S. market in 2001 due to increased risk of myopathy and rhabdomyolysis?
    A. Cerivastatin
    B. Cisapride
    C. Dexfenfluramine
    D. Terfenadine
    E. Astemizole

140. Doxycycline oral gel is used to treat
    A. periodontitis
    B. aphthous ulcers
    C. acne
    D. Lyme disease
    E. arthritis

141. Which of the following drugs requires a dosage adjustment in patients with renal impairment?
    A. Famotidine
    B. Capecitabine
    C. Gentamicin
    D. A and C
    E. A, B, and C

142. A prevalent side effect of norethindrone is
    A. diarrhea
    B. breakthrough bleeding
    C. blood dyscrasias
    D. cardiac insufficiency
    E. abortion

143. The preferred way to offset hypokalemia is to
    A. eat citrus fruits
    B. eat seafood or fish
    C. administer potassium salt
    D. administer IV electrolytes
    E. diminish urination

144. Persons receiving MAO inhibitors should control their intake of
    A. some fermented foods and beverages
    B. carbohydrates
    C. fats and lipids
    D. water
    E. salicylate analgesics

145. Which of the following drugs should **NOT** be administered with high-fat meals?
    I. Indinavir
    II. Riluzole
    III. Stavudine

    A. I only
    B. III only
    C. I and II only
    D. II and III only
    E. I, II, and III

146. Which of the following drugs may inhibit the metabolism of ziprasidone?
  I. Erythromycin
 II. Ketoconazole
III. Phenobarbital

  A. I only
  B. III only
  C. I and II only
  D. II and III only
  E. I, II, and III

147. Flumazenil is a specific antagonist for which of the following drugs?
  I. Meperidine
 II. Propoxyphene
III. Diazepam

  A. I only
  B. III only
  C. I and II only
  D. II and III only
  E. I, II, and III

148. Which of the following antidepressants also has an indication for smoking cessation?
  A. Haloperidol
  B. Bupropion
  C. Citalopram
  D. Mirtazapine
  E. Paroxetine

149. Docosanol is a (an)
  A. diuretic
  B. nonnarcotic analgesic
  C. anti-inflammatory
  D. antiviral
  E. anthelmintic

150. Which of the following statements is true regarding the administration of alendronate?

    I. Take more than 30 minutes before first food or beverage of the day

    II. Take with 6 to 8 ounces of plain water

    III. Remain fully upright (sitting or standing) for about 30 minutes

    A. I only
    B. III only
    C. I and II only
    D. II and III only
    E. I, II, and III

151. Testosterone is available as which of the following dosage forms?

    I. Ointment

    II. Injection

    III. Transdermal patch

    A. I only
    B. III only
    C. I and II only
    D. II and III only
    E. I, II, and III

152. Which of the following is an oral hypoglycemic agent?

    A. Ketorolac
    B. Pioglitazone
    C. Doconasol
    D. Riluzole
    E. Terbinafine

153. The concurrent administration (within 1 to 2 hours of dosing) of nislodipine should be avoided with which of the following?

    I. High-fat meal

    II. Grapefruit juice

    III. Cocoa

    A. I only
    B. III only

C. I and II only
D. II and III only
E. I, II, and III

154. Which of the following drugs may be administered without regard to meals?
   I. Valaciclovir
   II. Cetirizine
   III. Acarbose

   A. I only
   B. III only
   C. I and II only
   D. II and III only
   E. I, II, and III

155. Dexfenfluramine, an agent approved for the treatment of obesity, was removed from the U.S. market due to
   A. cardiac valvular dysfunction
   B. gastric ulcerations
   C. renal toxicity
   D. ototoxicity
   E. hepatic impairment

156. The terminal half-life of alendronate is
   A. 10 days
   B. 10 months
   C. 10 years
   D. 10 hours
   E. 10 minutes

157. Serotonin syndrome is characterized by which of the following symptoms?
   I. Mental status changes
   II. Tremor
   III. Diaphoresis

   A. I only
   B. III only
   C. I and II only
   D. II and III only
   E. I, II, and III

158. The FDA has recommended the removal of which ingredient found in cough/cold products due to an association with hemorrhagic stroke?

   A. Dextromethorphan
   B. Pseudoephedrine
   C. Guanfenisen
   D. Phenylpropanolamine
   E. Ephedrine

159. Which of the following antacids should not be used in dialysis patients?

   I. Aluminum hydroxide
   II. Magnesium hydroxide
   III. Calcium carbonate

   A. I only
   B. III only
   C. I and II only
   D. II and III only
   E. I, II, and III

160. Melatonin regulates which of the following functions?

   I. Sleep
   II. Circadian rhythms
   III. Respiration

   A. I only
   B. III only
   C. I and II only
   D. II and III only
   E. I, II, and III

161. Tacrolimus ointment is used primarily to treat

   A. pain
   B. atopic dermatitis
   C. sunburns
   D. skin grafts
   E. poison ivy

162. In 2001, which analgesic experienced significant misuses and diversion, requiring revisions in the warnings section of the product labeling?

A. OxyContin
B. Demerol
C. Tylenol #3
D. Toradol
E. Roxanol

163. Which of the following drug combinations has (have) been effective therapy for the treatment of *Helicobacter pylori*?
  I. Clarithromycin/ranitidine bismuth citrate
  II. Omeprazole/clarithromycin
  III. Ciprofloxacin/erythromycin

   A. I only
   B. III only
   C. I and II only
   D. II and III only
   E. I, II, and III

164. Ziprasidone, an agent used to treat schizophrenia, exerts its pharmacologic effects by
   A. inhibiting histamine reuptake
   B. stimulating serotonin synthesis
   C. blocking dopamine receptors
   D. stimulating dopamine release
   E. none of the above

165. Ocular timolol is used primarily to treat
   A. mydriasis
   B. glaucoma
   C. cataracts
   D. conjunctivitis
   E. none of the above

166. Cetirizine is a
   A. nonspecific histamine antagonist
   B. histamine 1 antagonist
   C. histamine 2 antagonist
   D. histamine 1 agonist
   E. histamine 2 agonist

167. Bivalirudin is a (an)
   A. anticoagulant
   B. anti-infective
   C. NSAID
   D. antiviral
   E. antihistamine

168. Cevimeline is used to treat
   A. dermatitis
   B. xerostomia
   C. allergic rhinitis
   D. tinea versicolor
   E. eczema

169. Crotalide is used to treat the bites of
   A. fleas
   B. North American vipers
   C. ticks
   D. rabid animals
   E. black widow spiders

170. Which of the following statements regarding fosphenytoin are true?
   I. Fosphenytoin is completely converted to phenytoin after intravenous or intramuscular administration
   II. The administration of 1 mmol of fosphenytoin produces 1 mmol of phenytoin
   III. Monitoring serum phenytoin levels is not necessary

   A. I only
   B. III only
   C. I and II only
   D. II and III only
   E. I, II, and III

171. Sumatriptan's efficacy in migraine therapy is attributed to which of the following mechanisms?
   I. Selective 5-HT(1) agonist
   II. Nonspecific 5-HT agonist
   III. Dopamine agonist

A. I only
B. III only
C. I and II only
D. II and III only
E. I, II, and III

172. The principal adverse effect of acarbose is
    A. hematologic
    B. gastrointestinal
    C. renal
    D. hepatic
    E. dermal

173. Unoprostone is FDA approved to treat
    A. ovarian cancer
    B. Hodgkin's disease
    C. open angle glaucoma
    D. conjunctivitis
    E. tinnitus

174. Oral or parenteral ketorolac therapy is limited to 5 days of therapy due to an increased risk of
    A. renal impairment
    B. gastrointestinal bleeding/perforation
    C. liver failure
    D. CNS disturbances
    E. A and B

175. Which of the following HMG-CoA reductase inhibitors causes the greatest percentage increase in HDL?
    A. Simvastatin
    B. Pravastatin
    C. Lovastatin
    D. Fluvastatin
    E. All produce equivalent reductions

176. Sibutramine should not be used in patients
 I. with a body mass index greater than 30 kg/m²
 II. taking MAO inhibitors
 III. with poorly controlled hypertension

 A. I only
 B. III only
 C. I and II only
 D. II and III only
 E. I, II, and III

177. Which of the following statement(s) regarding low-molecular-weight heparins (LMWHs) is (are) true?
 I. Predominantly inhibits thrombin
 II. Does not require APTT monitoring
 III. Has a stronger affinity than conventional heparin for factor II

 A. I only
 B. III only
 C. I and II only
 D. II and III only
 E. I, II, and III

178. Which of the following statements is true regarding indinavir?
 I. It prevents the production of infectious virus in infected cells
 II. It competitively inhibits the HIV protease enzyme
 III. It is a reverse transcriptase inhibitor

 A. I only
 B. III only
 C. I and II only
 D. II and III only
 E. I, II, and III

179. Diuretics tend to enhance lithium salt toxicity due to
 A. sodium depletion
 B. potassium depletion
 C. direct drug interaction

    D. increased absorption

    E. increased solubility of the lithium salts

180. Leflunomide is used to treat

    A. Crohn's disease

    B. rheumatoid arthritis

    C. psoriasis

    D. photoallergic reaction

    E. none of the above

181. Sumatriptan use is contraindicated in patients

    I. with a history of ischemic heart disease

   II. taking phenelzine

  III. with uncontrolled hypertension

    A. I only

    B. III only

    C. I and II only

    D. II and III only

    E. I, II, and III

182. Eptifibatide is classified as a (an)

    A. fluoroquinolone

    B. glycoprotein IIb/IIIa receptor inhibitor

    C. diuretic

    D. antihypertensive

    E. none of the above

183. Finasteride's action in the treatment of benign prostatic hypertrophy is as a (an)

    A. HMG-CoA reductase inhibitor

    B. alpha-5 reductase inhibitor

    C. serotonin reuptake inhibitor

    D. P450 hepatic enzyme inhibitor

    E. none of the above

184. A useful agent in the treatment of bladder incontinence is

    A. nalmefene

    B. tolterodine

    C. tolcapone

    D. valrubicin

    E. none of the above

185. Which of the following agents are approved for treatment of narcolepsy?
   I. Modafinil
   II. Methylphenidate
   III. Dextroamphetamine

   A. I only
   B. III only
   C. I and II only
   D. II and III only
   E. I, II, and III

186. Misoprostol is used to
   A. treat gastric ulcers
   B. prevent NSAID-induced gastric ulcers
   C. prevent osteoporosis
   D. prevent renal toxicity
   E. treat Paget's disease

187. The combination of use of metformin and iodinated contrast media are contraindicated because it increases the risk of
   A. hypertension
   B. CNS depression
   C. allergic reactions
   D. lactic acidosis
   E. hypoglycemia

188. Acarbose, a hypoglycemic agent, exerts which of the following mechanisms of action?
   A. Increases insulin secretion
   B. Increases insulin receptor sensitivity
   C. Decreases circulating insulin antibodies
   D. Delays digestion of carbohydrates
   E. None of the above

189. Which of the following drugs interferes with the metabolism of indinavir?
   A. Ketoconazole
   B. Ciprofloxacin
   C. Digoxin
   D. Lorazepam
   E. None of the above

190. Which of the following adverse drug effects have been associated with isotretinoin use?

   I. Suicidal ideation
  II. Teratogenecity
 III. Hypertriglyceridemia

  A. I only
  B. III only
  C. I and II only
  D. II and III only
  E. I, II, and III

191. How does rifampin decrease the efficacy of certain oral contraceptives?

  A. Increases oral contraceptive renal clearance
  B. Increases oral contraceptive metabolism via hepatic enzyme induction
  C. Reduces oral contraceptive systemic circulation via protein binding
  D. Decreases intestinal absorption of oral contraceptives
  E. None of the above

192. Fexofenadine is a

  A. metabolite of loratadine
  B. metabolite of astemizole
  C. metabolite of terfenadine
  D. metabolite of hydroxyzine
  E. none of the above

193. Levetiracetam is considered a (an)

  A. antianxiety agent
  B. benzodiazepine
  C. anticonvulsant
  D. antihistamine
  E. antineoplastic

194. Which mechanism(s) of action is (are) responsible for suc-
cimer's efficacy in the treatment of lead poisoning?
   I. Increases the renal excretion of lead
   II. Chelates lead into water soluble complexes
   III. Promotes lead degradation to nontoxic metabolites

   A. I only
   B. III only
   C. I and II only
   D. II and III only
   E. I, II, and III

195. The advantages of transdermal estrogens as compared to
oral estrogens when used for estrogen replacement therapy
include
   I. less frequent dosing
   II. increased cardioprotection
   III. decreased incidence of thrombolic events

   A. I only
   B. III only
   C. I and II only
   D. II and III only
   E. I, II, and III

196. Mirtazapine is a potent antagonist of
   A. 5-HT(2) receptors
   B. 5-HT(3) receptors
   C. 5-HT(1) receptors
   D. A and B
   E. none of the above

197. Which of the following activities is (are) responsible for
prominent sedative effects?
   I. Histamine-1 receptor antagonism
   II. Increased melatonin secretion
   III. Dopamine receptor antagonism

   A. I only
   B. III only
   C. I and II only

D. II and III only
E. I, II, and III

198. A combination of an antiretroviral and a protease inhibitor may result in which of the following actions?
   I. Sustained reduction in viral load
   II. Decrease the development of resistance
   III. Reduce the incidence of opportunistic infections

   A. I only
   B. III only
   C. I and II only
   D. II and III only
   E. I, II, and III

199. Naratriptan is useful in the treatment of acute migraine via its action as a
   A. serotonin agonist
   B. serotonin antagonist
   C. histamine antagonist
   D. histamine inhibitor
   E. prostaglandin inhibitor

200. Which of the following drugs has an FDA pregnancy category X rating?
   A. Lorazepam
   B. Warfarin
   C. Penicillin
   D. Isotretinoin
   E. Metaproterenol

201. Cystic fibrosis patients routinely need supplementation with
   A. fat-soluble vitamins
   B. carbohydrates
   C. mannitol
   D. water-soluble vitamins
   E. none of the above

202. Immune globulin is administered parenterally to provide passive immunity to patients with which of the following disease states?
A. Bone marrow transplant
B. Idiopathic thrombocytopenic purpura
C. AIDS
D. Kawasaki syndrome
E. All of the above

203. There are many pancreatic enzyme preparations on the U.S. market. To therapeutically substitute these products in a cystic fibrosis patient, the _____ portion should be equivalent doses.
A. amylase
B. protease
C. trypsinogen
D. lipase
E. trypsin

204. All of the following are effective in the treatment of acute gouty arthritis, EXCEPT
A. colchicine
B. indomethacin
C. corticosteroids
D. NSAIDs
E. allopurinol

205. Signs and symptoms of theophylline toxicity include
A. sinus tachycardia
B. insomnia
C. seizures
D. nausea/vomiting
E. all of the above

206. Insulin resistance is often due to
A. excessive exercise
B. upper body obesity
C. acute renal failure
D. B and C
E. A, B, and C

207. Side effects associated with oral iron therapy include
  A. constipation
  B. diarrhea
  C. dark stools
  D. nausea
  E. all of the above

208. Diarrhea is a side effect **COMMONLY** associated with which of the following drugs?
  A. Codeine
  B. Quinidine
  C. Procainamide
  D. Acetaminophen
  E. Amitriptyline

209. Which of the following can be used to treat constipation or chronic, watery diarrhea?
  A. Hyperosmolar laxatives
  B. Bulk-forming laxatives
  C. Saline laxatives
  D. Stimulant laxatives
  E. All of the above

210. Ergot alkaloids are contraindicated for use in patients with
  A. venous insufficiency
  B. ischemic heart disease
  C. sepsis
  D. pregnancy
  E. all of the above

211. Which of the following erythromycin salts has been associated with cholestasis?
  A. Ethylsuccinate
  B. Gluceptate
  C. Lactobionate
  D. Stearate
  E. Estolate

212. Anticholinergic agents may aggravate which of the following?
   A. Narrow angle glaucoma
   B. GI obstruction
   C. Genitourinary tract disease
   D. Severe cardiac disease
   E. All of the above

213. Side effects of heparin include
   A. thrombocytopenia
   B. gingivitis
   C. glaucoma
   D. hyperglycemia
   E. none of the above

214. Which of the following drugs may interact with digoxin?
   A. Quinidine
   B. Antacids
   C. Cholestyramine
   D. A and B
   E. A, B, and C

215. Which of the following drugs interferes with theophylline?
   A. Cimetidine
   B. Erythromycin
   C. Ciprofloxacin
   D. Oral contraceptives
   E. All of the above

Pharmacology

Answers and Discussion

1. **(B)** Etanercept, a tumor necrosis factor inhibitor, was approved by the FDA in 1998 for the treatment of rheumatoid arthritis.

2. **(A)** Dosage is regularly adjusted upward if attacks occur frequently.

3. **(D)** If arrest occurs, it is due to asystole.

4. **(A)** The conjugation is primarily by acetylation.

5. **(A)** Tinnitus is a common sign of salicylate toxicity and represents blood salicylate levels reaching or exceeding the upper limits of therapeutic ranges. Temporary hearing loss disappears gradually upon discontinuation of the drug.

6. **(A)** The disease is characterized by low levels of brain dopamine.

7. **(C)** Medullary paralysis can occur with overdoses.

8. **(C)** Nalorphine is structurally similar to morphine derivatives and has some agonistic activity.

9. **(A)** Allopurinol interferes with uric acid synthesis and is a good prophylactic agent to prevent gout.

10. **(B)** Colesevelam is an oral bile acid sequestrate approved by the FDA in 2000 for the reduction of low-density lipoproteins.

11. **(D)** A deficiency of vitamin B_1 produces beriberi.

12. **(D)** Capecitabine is an oral antineoplastic approved by the FDA in 1998 for the treatment of metastatic breast cancer.

13. **(D)** Magnesium ion plays an important role in all of the activities listed.

14. **(D)** Many of the migraine drugs are ergot derivatives.

15. **(E)** All are potential complications of enteral feedings.

16. **(B)** Leucovorin (folinic acid), the formyl derivative and active form of folic acid, is considered an antidote for folic acid antagonists, such as methotrexate (>100 mg/m^2) or trimethoprim.

17. **(C)** Cyclosporine is an immunosuppressive agent that has low toxicity.

18. **(A)** Pantoprazole is a proton pump inhibitor that prevents gastric acid secretion and was approved by the FDA in 2000 for the short-term treatment of erosive esophagitis.

19. **(C)** Citalopram, is an oral selective serotonin reuptake inhibitor, which was approved by the FDA in 1998 for the treatment of depression.

20. **(B)** For daunorubicin, myocardial toxicity, as potentially fatal congestive heart failure, may occur when a total cumulative dosage exceeds 400 to 550 mg/m^2 in adults, 300 mg/m^2 in children over 2, or 10 mg/kg in children under 2. This effect may occur during therapy or within several months to years after therapy. For doxorubicin, the risk of

developing congestive heart failure increases with increasing total cumulative dose in excess of 450 mg/m^2. Such toxicity may occur at lower doses in patients with predisposing factors (e.g., chest irradiation).

21. **(E)** Nicotine is available as a nonprescription product either as an ion-exchange resin in a sugar-free chewing gum base or as a transdermal patch. As a prescription product nicotine is available both as a nasal spray and an oral inhaler (Nicotrol Inhaler or Nicotrol NS).

22. **(E)** Triamcinolone produces all the side effects of the class (including depression, water retention, effects on blood sugar, and increasing susceptibility to infection), but does not increase appetite.

23. **(E)** Propylthiouracil inhibits the *synthesis* of thyroid hormones. However, if thyroid hormones are already present, propylthiouracil will not inhibit their action. This is the case whether the thyroid hormones were produced naturally or administered exogenously.

24. **(A)** Approximately 2,500 to 3,000 U.S. infants are born annually with spina bifida or anencephaly (known as neural tube defects) caused by the incomplete closing of the spine and skull. In 1998, the Food and Nutrition Board of the National Academy of Sciences Institute of Medicine (IOM) recommended that to reduce the risk for neural tube defects, women capable of becoming pregnant should take 400 µg of synthetic folic acid daily, from fortified foods or supplements or a combination of the two, in addition to consuming folate in a varied diet.

25. **(D)** Even the administration of a single thalidomide tablet during pregnancy has been associated with severe birth defects. Thus, in the United States the distribution of this drug is limited to a special restricted distribution program known as S.T.E.P.S. (System for Thalidomide Education and Prescribing Safety). Only prescribers and pharmacists registered and trained via the program are allowed to prescribe and dispense the product.

26. (B) Peripheral neuropathy associated with isoniazid administration is most likely due to interference with pyridoxine metabolism. Thus, in persons with conditions where neuropathy may be common (e.g., diabetes, uremia, malnutrition), the administration of pyridoxine is recommended. Recommended prophylactic doses range from 6 to 100 mg/d.

27. (A) The only advantage is that amoxicillin is not easily destroyed by stomach acid.

28. (E) Balsalazide, an oral prodrug of mesalamine, was approved by the FDA in 2000 for the treatment of mild to moderate active ulcerative colitis.

29. (A) Arsenic trioxide is an antineoplastic arsenical compound approved to treat acute promyelocytic leukemia.

30. (B) Primidone is a deoxybarbiturate which is metabolized to two active metabolites, phenylethylmalonamide (PEMA) and phenobarbital. Serum concentrations of phenobarbital are used to monitor patients taking primidone.

31. (A) One of the dose-limiting effects of vincristine is the neurotoxic effects of the drug. Peripheral neuropathy may present as tingling and numbness in the feet.

32. (B) Oral or parenteral dolasetron is used to treat or prevent emesis associated with cancer chemotherapy.

33. (D) Botulinum toxin A was initially FDA approved for the treatment of strabismus and blepharospasms in patients at least 12 years old. In 2000, botulinum toxin B was approved for the treatment of cervical dystonias. Because the agent causes temporary local paralysis of muscles at the site of injection, it is also used for the reduction of facial wrinkles as an off-label indication.

34. (D) It is a semisynthetic tetracycline given every 12 hours.

35. (A) Cholestyramine resin has an affinity for bile salts and interferes with absorption of fat. Fat-soluble vitamins may not be absorbed. It reduces cholesterol levels and has none of the other effects listed.

36. **(B)** All have diuretic activity except glyburide, which is an oral antidiabetic agent.

37. **(E)** All are true. Tetracyclines are quite readily absorbed.

38. **(E)** Gatifloxacin, a fluoroquinolone, was approved by the FDA in 1999.

39. **(D)** Infliximab is a chimeric monoclonal antibody that was approved by the FDA in 1998 and is indicated for the treatment of rheumatoid arthritis and Crohn's disease.

40. **(D)** Because it produces sedation, loss of memory, and reduction of anxiety, lorazepam is used as a preoperative medication.

41. **(E)** Celecoxib, a cyclo-oxygenase-2 inhibitor, was FDA approved in 1998 for the treatment of osteoarthritis and rheumatoid arthritis. It has analgesic and anti-inflammatory effects.

42. **(A)** Timolide is a combination of timolol maleate and the diuretic hydrochlorothiazide, used to treat hypertension.

43. **(A)** The use of salicylates during certain viral illnesses (e.g., influenza A, influenza B and varicella) may be a factor in the pathogenesis of Reye's syndrome. The Centers for Disease Control advises caution in administering salicylates to children with a viral illness.

44. **(E)** The rapid action and short duration of action make ultra–short-acting barbiturates ideal for inducing anesthesia.

45. **(B)** Norethindrone has both progestational activity and mild estrogenic activity, and is widely used in oral contraceptives.

46. **(B)** Carbamazepine, phenytoin, or gabapentin have been used as off-label indications to treat diabetic neuropathy, trigeminal neuralgias, or peripheral neuropathy.

47. (E) The principal action of this drug is as a non-nucleoside reverse transcriptase inhibitor and was FDA approved in 1998 for the treatment of HIV-1 infection.

48. (C) Lepirudin, a hirudin analog anticoagulant, was FDA approved in 1998 for the treatment of heparin-induced thrombocytopenia.

49. (E) Histamine is found at all three sites.

50. (C) Orlistat, a reversible lipase inhibitor, was approved by the FDA in 1999 for the management of obesity.

51. (C) Codeine may cause constipation rather than diarrhea.

52. (C) Antipsychotics produce calmness without sedation, hypnosis, motor impairment, or euphoria.

53. (D) Lidocaine is used as a local anesthetic and for ventricular arrhythmias.

54. (D) Cocaine is a vasoconstrictor and prevents its own absorption, keeping the drug localized longer.

55. (B) Diethylstilbestrol was the first synthetic estrogen introduced.

56. (D) Propylthiouracil is an antithyroid agent. The others are thyroid hormones and are contraindicated in hyperthyroidism.

57. (C) Carbidopa has no therapeutic activity, but prevents degradation of L-dopa.

58. (A) Hyoscyamine is the levo isomer of the racemic mixture known as atropine. The dextro isomer is almost inactive.

59. (D) Gemtuzumab is a cytotoxic antitumor antibiotic approved by the FDA in 2000 to treat refractory or relapsed acute myeloid leukemia.

60. (A) All side effects are seen, but hemorrhage is the principal one, usually due to overdosage.

61. (B) Tenecteplase is a plasminogen activator thrombolytic approved in 2000 for the reduction of mortality associated with acute myocardial infarction.

62. (C) Albuterol is much more effective in treating bronchospasm when given by inhalation. Oral forms are used less frequently.

63. (C) Nateglinide was approved in 2000 to treat type II diabetes.

64. (B) They are among the most potent of the enzyme inducers.

65. (A) Meloxicam is a nonsteroidal anti-inflammatory agent approved in 2000 for the treatment of osteoarthritis.

66. (A) Penicillins act primarily by inhibition of cell wall synthesis in susceptible microorganisms, and are bacteriocidal.

67. (E) All three effects are seen; epinephrine is poorly effective when administered orally.

68. (D) Amrinone is a synthetic bipyridine derivative. Nitroglycerin is not a cardiac glycoside. The others occur naturally.

69. (A) Oxcarbazepine is a prodrug of carbamazepine and was approved in 2000 for the treatment of partial seizures in epileptic adults and children aged 4 to 16 years.

70. (C) Atropine is the prototypical cholinergic antagonist. The others are cholinergic agonists.

71. (E) Protamine sulfate quickly terminates the action of heparin on a 1:1 mole basis.

72. (D) Although nitroglycerin is volatile and somewhat unstable, its short half-life is due to metabolic instability caused by extensive first-pass metabolism.

73. **(B)** Various opiates are used as analgesics, antitussives, and antidiarrheals, and to induce anesthesia. However, they exhibit no significant anti-inflammatory activity.

74. **(A)** Trihexylphenidyl is related to atropine and is used primarily to treat parkinsonism.

75. **(D)** Antihistaminics compete for the same receptor sites with histamine.

76. **(E)** Isotretinoin is closely related to vitamin A and is used to treat acne.

77. **(A)** Endorphins are released in times of stress and have a marked role in pain perception.

78. **(E)** Colchicine gives immediate and most effective relief from the pain of gout. Other drugs are slower in activity. Para-aminobenzoic acid (PABA) is not used to treat gout.

79. **(C)** Nystatin is very effective against *Candida* infestations, but is ineffective against *Trichomonas,* bacteria, and rickettsia.

80. **(B)** Ketorolac is available both orally and parenterally. The manufacturer recommends that the total duration of therapy (both oral and parenteral) is indicated for short-term (not to exceed 5 days) management of moderately severe acute pain requiring analgesia at the opioid level.

81. **(C)** Musculoskeletal pain is usually of short duration; specific therapy for longer periods is unwarranted.

82. **(A)** Linezolid was FDA approved in 2000 for the treatment of vancomycin-resistant *Enterococcus faecium* (VRE) infection and nosocomial pneumonia caused by *Staphylococcus aureus* including MRSA or *Streptococcus penumoniae.*

83. **(A)** Nateglinide is used as an adjunct to metformin for control of hyperglycemia in patients with type II diabetes.

84. (E) Mifeprostone is an oral abortifacient that acts as a progesterone receptor antagonist.

85. (A) Rivastigmine is a reversible carbamate acetylcholinesterase inhibitor that interacts preferentially with acetylcholinesterase G, which is found in high levels in the brains of patients with Alzheimer's disease. The inhibition lasts for 10 hours.

86. (E) All of these agents are low-molecular-weight heparins.

87. (A) Timolol is a nonselective β-adrenergic blocking agent that lowers intraocular pressure.

88. (A) Sucralfate exerts local activity in healing ulcers only.

89. (D) Lorazepam is a member of the dibenzazepine class and is used to treat anxiety.

90. (E) Because probantheline is an anticholinergic drug, it is contraindicated in all of the conditions listed.

91. (C) Because of long-term and regular usage, antiepileptics as a group cause development of tolerance; alternating therapy is commonly used.

92. (B) Selenium sulfide is far too toxic for systemic use, but is used topically as an antifungal, antibacterial, or keratolytic agent.

93. (B) Zonisamide is an anticonvulsant approved by the FDA in 2000 for the adjunct treatment of partial seizures in adults.

94. (E) All are stimulant-type laxatives except docusate, which is a stool softener.

95. (A) Sympathomimetics cause all of the listed actions except that they dilate the pupil of the eye.

96. (C) Baclofen is a centrally acting muscle relaxant. It is not indicated in anxiety or tension problems.

97. (D) Beta-interferon is effective in slowing the progression of multiple sclerosis.

98. (D) Propylthiouracil may cause agranulocytopenia, leukopenia, or dermatitis.

99. (B) Candesartan, an angiotensin II receptor antagonist, was approved in 1998 for treatment of hypertension.

100. (E) Sulindac exhibits all these pharmacologic activities.

101. (A) Mirtazapine is an antidepressant that acts via serotonin inhibition.

102. (C) Ofloxacin is effective against a broad variety of gram-positive and gram-negative bacteria; it is not effective against fungi, rickettsia, or virus infections.

103. (D) Zidovudine interferes with maturation of red blood cells and may cause or exacerbate anemia. It tends to cause vasodilation and CNS depression less frequently.

104. (C) Mupirocin is produced by *Pseudomonas fluorescens* and is used to treat impetigo. It may not be used in the eye or on other mucous membranes.

105. (B) Pentoxifylline thins blood and is useful in occlusive arterial disease of the skin. It has no effect on cholesterol or biotransformation.

106. (A) Sodium nitroprusside gives immediate and dramatic lowering of blood pressure. The other agents are used in milder hypertensions or to relieve edema.

107. (B) Most agents increase elimination of uric acid. Allopurinol prevents formation and acts more slowly to lower uric acid levels.

108. (A) This is particularly true in postmenopausal women. Estrogens also should not be used during pregnancy because of their risk to offspring.

109. (B) Because of the potential for excessive hypotensive effects as a result of increased cGMP, the concomitant use of sildenafil and organic nitrates is contraindicated.

110. (D) Gentamicin is noted for nephrotoxicity, as is true of other aminoglycoside antibiotics.

111. (B) Risendronate is a bisphosphonate that was FDA approved in 1998 for the treatment of Paget's disease.

112. (E) Carbamazepine has been found to be effective in trigeminal neuralgia; however, it is not a simple analgesic, and should not be used for more trivial pain.

113. (B) Although methylphenidate is a relatively mild CNS stimulant, it is recommended only for attention deficit disorders.

114. (E) Doxorubicin is a potent and dangerous cytotoxic agent used primarily to treat hematologic malignancies and solid tumors.

115. (C) Amphotericin B is often effective in potentially fatal fungus infestations. The other antifungals listed are not as potent.

116. (B) Thyroid hormones have been shown to be ineffective either alone or in combination with other agents.

117. (D) Dextromethorphan is only about half as effective as codeine; however, it has no analgesic activity and little CNS depression.

118. (A) Nonselective 2-adrenoreceptor antagonists are used for such conditions as frostbite, phlebitis, and Raynaud's disease. They are contraindicated in atherosclerosis and renal insufficiency.

119. (E) It is a nonselective beta antagonist.

120. (E) Antimuscarinics are contraindicated in all three, plus achalasia of the esophagus and bladder niche obstruction.

121. (D) Both drugs were approved in 1999 for the treatment of influenza A and B infections. Only osteltamivir is approved for prophylaxis.

122. (D) Sulfisoxazole is a sulfonamide derivative most often used in combination with trimethoprim for the treatment of bacterial infections, such as UTIs or otitis media.

123. (E) Lens opacity may occur after prolonged use; other eye problems are quite uncommon.

124. (A) Furosemide increases the toxicity of digitalis.

125. (D) Progestins frequently stimulate diarrhea; they are not constipating.

126. (E) All of these drugs carry a risk of QTc interval prolongation and require baseline ECG prior to initiation of therapy.

127. (C) Lamivudine, an antiviral agent, was approved in 1998 for the treatment of hepatitis B infections.

128. (D) Nitrates such as amylnitrate or nitroglycerin are notorious for developing tolerance.

129. (A) Streptokinase is produced by hemolytic streptococci and is capable of dissolving blood clots. It is particularly useful to dissolve pulmonary clots.

130. (D) Gold compounds alter the properties of collagen and inhibit phagocytosis.

131. (B) Tamoxifen is a potent antiestrogen used to treat metastatic breast cancer.

132. (E) Bacitracin is highly nephrotoxic and is rarely used parenterally. Its major use is for topical application.

133. (B) Thiamine is necessary for normalization of cardiovascular and neurologic symptoms; beriberi may result from a deficiency of this vitamin.

134. (A) Librium shows a cross-dependence with alcohol and is effective. Antabuse is used only as a preventative to drinking.

135. (D) Cromolyn is not effective if histamine is released, but it does prevent release from mast cells.

136. (E) Aspirin inhibits synthesis of prostaglandins, which mediate inflammation.

137. (C) Ricinoleic acid is formed by the hydrolysis of pancreatic lipases and is a powerful irritant.

138. (B) Penicillamine is a chelating agent that ties up copper deposits typically found in Wilson's disease.

139. (A) In August 2001, cerivastatin was removed from the U.S. market based on repeated postmarketing surveillance reports of rhabdomyolysis and myopathy when used alone or in combination of gemfibrozil. Cisapride was withdrawn in 2000 due to QT prolongation. Dexfenfluramine was withdrawn in 1997 due to aortic and mitral regurgitation. Terfenadine was withdrawn in 1998 and astemizole with drawn in 1999, both related to reports of cardiac arrhythmias.

140. (A) Doxycycline oral gel was marketed in 1998 as therapy for periodontitis.

141. (E) All these drugs require dosage adjustments in patients with renal impairment. Famotidine dosages should be reduced in patients with moderate to severe renal impairment ($Cr_{cl} < 50$ mL/min). Capecitabine should be reduced to 75% of recommended normal doses in patient with mild renal impairment. Gentamicin requires adjustment in dosage intervals in renal impairment.

142. (B) Norethindrone is usually used in combinations to decrease breakthrough bleeding.

143. (A) Citrus fruits are rich in potassium and represent the preferred approach to lessen the tendency for other problems.

144. (A) Many fermented foods and beverages contain tyramine, which can be toxic if not destroyed by monoamine oxidase.

145. (C) When administered with a high-fat meal, indinavir's AUC is reduced by 77% and C_{max} is reduced by 84%; riluzole's AUC is reduced by 20% and its C_{max} is reduced by 45%. These products should be administered 1 hour before or 2 hours after meals. Stavudine may be administered without regard to meals.

146. (C) Ziprasidone is metabolized by the cytochrome P450 isoenzyme (CYP3A4) system. Thus, drugs that are specific CYP3A4 inhibitors interfere with its metabolism. Both erythromycin and ketoconazole are CYP3A4 inhibitors. Phenobarbital is a CYP3A4 inducer.

147. (B) Flumazenil is a benzodiazepine receptor antagonist. It obstructs the actions of benzodiazepines on the CNS and competitively inhibits the activity on the GABA benzodiazepine receptor complex.

148. (B) Bupropion is indicated for the treatment of depression as Wellbutrin and for smoking cessation as Zyban.

149. (D) Docosanol is a topical antiviral indicated for the treatment of cold sores and fever blisters. This agent was approved in 2000 by the FDA.

150. (E) All three statements are true. The bioavailability of this drug after oral administration is poor and may be reduced by several factors. Noncompliance with these administration guidelines has resulted in esophagitis and/or gastrointestinal ulceration.

151. (E) Testosterone is available in all three dosage forms: The patch and injection are indicated for replacement therapy in males for conditions associated with deficiency or absence of endogenous testosterone. Certain injections are also used in women with inoperable breast cancers. The ointment is used for vulvar dystrophy.

152. (B) Pioglitazone is an oral hypoglycemic agent approved in 1999 as an adjunct to diet and exercise or in combination with insulin, sulfonylurea, or metformin to lower blood glucose in patients with type II diabetes.

153. (C) Nislodipine bioavailability (AUC) may be reduced by approximately 20% when administered within 1 to 2 hours of grapefruit juice products. Administration with a high-fat meal may lead to excessive peak concentrations (300%).

154. (C) Valciclovir and cetirizine bioavailability are unaffected by concurrent food administration. Acarbose should be administered three times daily with the first bite of each main meal.

155. (A) Dexfenfluramine is a serotonin agonist that promotes the release and inhibits the reuptake of serotonin in the CNS. Dexfenfluramine was withdrawn in 1997 due to aortic and mitral regurgitation.

156. (C) The half-life of alendronate in humans is greater than 10 years, reflecting its slow release from the skeleton.

157. (E) The serotonin syndrome results from increased CNS serotonin levels and usually results from an overdose of a serotonergic agent or concurrent therapy with two serotonergic drugs. All of these symptoms reflect increased serotonin levels.

158. (D) In November 2000, the FDA recommended the removal of phenylpropanolamine from over-the-counter diet aids and cough/cold products based on a retrospective study that associated use with a risk of hemorrhagic stroke.

159. (C) In dialysis patients the excretion of aluminum and magnesium is decreased, resulting in toxic accumulation. Calcium carbonate may be used to bind phosphate in dialysis patients.

160. (C) Melatonin, an endogenous hormone secreted by the pineal gland, is available commercially as a nutritional supplement for various purposes. Endogenous secretion of melatonin aids in the regulation of sleep and circadian rhythm.

161. (B) Topical tacrolimus is used to treat atopic dermatitis.

162. (A) In July 2001, FDA and Purdue Pharmaceuticals strengthened the warnings and precautions sections in the labeling of OxyContin, a narcotic drug approved for the treatment of moderate to severe pain, because of continuing reports of abuse and diversion. The changes were intended to reinforce proper prescription practices and increase physician focus on the potential for abuse, misuse, and diversion.

163. (C) Clarithromycin with ranitidine is commercially available as a combination tablet to treat *H pylori*. Omeprazole with clarithromycin has also been a successful combination in the treatment of *H pylori*.

164. (C) Ziprasidone is an atypical antipsychotic which is a serotonin (5HT)-ZA-dopamine antagonist.

165. (B) Ocular timolol is effective in lowering intraocular pressure in chronic open angle glaucoma.

166. (B) Cetirizine is a specific histamine 1 antagonist approved for the treatment of allergic rhinitis.

167. (A) Bivalirudin is an anticoagulant that the FDA approved in 2000 for the prevention of clotting associated with percutaneous transluminal coronary angioplasty.

168. (B) Cevimeline is an oral muscarinic agent used to treat xerostomia associated with Sjögren's syndrome.

169. (B) Crotalide was marketed in 2000 as antivenin for North American viper bites.

170. (C) Fosphenytoin is a prodrug of phenytoin that is completely converted to phenytoin after parenteral administration with a 1:1 mmol equivalency. The conversion half-life of fosphenytoin to phenytoin is 15 minutes. It is recommended that phenytoin plasma concentrations not be monitored until conversion to phenytoin is complete.

171. **(A)** Sumatriptan is a selective agonist for vascular 5-HT(1) receptor and has no significant activity at 5-HT(2) or 5-HT(3) receptor subtypes or at dopamine, alpha 1, alpha 2, or beta-adrenergic receptors.

172. **(B)** Acarbose, an alpha-glucosidase inhibitor, acts locally in the GI tract to delay the digestion of carbohydrates and thus delay glucose absorption and lower postprandial glucose levels. Thus, the most commonly cited side effects are local and GI in nature, including flatulence (77%) and diarrhea (33%).

173. **(C)** Unoprostone, a prostaglandin F2-alpha analog, was FDA approved in 2000 to lower ocular pressure in open angle glaucoma.

174. **(E)** Ketorolac inhibits platelet function, and with continued use (>5 days) may increase the risk of GI bleeding/perforation and has also been associated with changes in renal function.

175. **(E)** HDL may be increased by all statins, simvastatin (5% to 21%), lovastatin (7% to 10%), pravastatin (4% to 8%), and fluvastatin (3% to 8%).

176. **(D)** Sibutramine is contraindicated for use with MAOIs and in patients diagnosed with poorly controlled hypertension.

177. **(C)** LMWHs range in mass from 3000 to 800 daltons, have a lower affinity for heparin cofactor II, and their efficacy in the treatment of deep vein thrombosis does not correlate with activated partial thromboplastin time (APTT).

178. **(B)** Indinavir inhibits HIV protease, the enzyme required for proteolytic cleavage of the viral polyprotein precursors into individual functional proteins, thus forming immature

noninfecting viral particles. This agent influences viral production in already infected cells.

179. (A) Diuretics decrease resorption of sodium and hence increase concentration of lithium.

180. (B) Leflunomide was approved for the management of rheumatoid arthritis in 1998 by the FDA.

181. (E) IV sumatriptan has the potential to cause coronary vasospasm and/or increases in blood pressure and thus is contraindicated for use in patients with a history of angina, myocardial infarctions (MI), ischemic disease, or uncontrolled hypertension. This agent also should not be used concurrently with or within 2 weeks of discontinuing an MAOI because it can increase sumatriptan AUC and half-life.

182. (B) Eptifibatide, a glycoprotein IIb/IIIa receptor inhibitor, was FDA approved in 1998 for the use in acute coronary syndrome.

183. (B) Finasteride inhibits 5-alpha reductase, the enzyme that converts testosterone into 5-alpha dihydrotestosterone (DHT). DHT is responsible for prostate gland development.

184. (B) Tolterodine was FDA approved to manage an overactive bladder. Tolcapone is indicated as adjunctive therapy for Parkinson's disease. Valrubicin is an antineoplastic administered intravesically for BCG refractory carcinoma in situ.

185. (E) All agents are approved for the management of narcolepsy.

186. (B) Misoprostol is used in combination with NSAIDs to prevent gastric ulcers.

187. (D) Metformin therapy should be withheld for at least 48 hours prior to and 48 hours subsequent to a procedure using iodinated contrast media and only restarted after renal function has been reevaluated and found to be normal. Several cases of lactic acidosis have been reported in patients receiving metformin and undergoing a procedure using iodinated contrast media.

188. (D) Acarbose, an alpha-glucosidase inhibitor, acts locally in the gastrointestinal tract to delay the digestion of carbohydrates, thus delaying glucose absorption and lowering postprandial glucose levels.

189. (A) A dose reduction of indinavir should be considered when administered with ketoconazole; ketoconazole increases the AUC by approximately 70%.

190. (E) Suicidal ideation, teratogenecity, and hypertriglyceridemia are known risks associated with isotretinoin therapy.

191. (B) Rifampin decreases the metabolism of oral contraceptives by inducing hepatic enzyme induction and reducing circulating estrogen levels.

192. (C) Fexofenadine is a metabolite of terfenadine with selective peripheral histamine-1 blocking activity. It is indicated for the relief of symptoms associated with seasonal allergic rhinitis in adults and children (>12 years).

193. (C) Levetiracetam was approved in 1999 as adjunctive therapy in the treatment of partial onset seizures in adults.

194. (C) Succimer, an analog of dimercaprol, forms water-soluble chelates of heavy metals, which are subsequently excreted renally.

195. (A) Transdermal estrogen therapy offers less frequent dosing when compared to oral therapy, but does not increase cardioprotection or affect the incidence of thrombotic events.

196. (D) Mirtazapine, an antidepressant with a tetracyclic chemical structure unrelated to other compounds, is a potent antagonist of 5-HT(2) and 5-HT(3) receptors. It has no significant activity for 5-HT(1) receptors.

197. (C) Increased melatonin secretion and antihistaminic effects at the 1 receptor site are associated with clinical symptoms of sedation.

198. (C) The combination of antiretrovirals and a protease inhibitor offers a sustained reduction in viral load and a delay or decrease in the development of resistance to either agent. The effect of this combination on the development of opportunistic infections is unknown.

199. (A) Naratriptan is considered a serotonin agonist and is used in the treatment of acute migraines with or without auras.

200. (D) Isotretinoin has an FDA pregnancy category X rating.

201. (A) Cystic fibrosis patients lack pancreatic digestive enzymes. Due to lipase deficiency, the fat-soluble vitamins are not well absorbed and are therefore commonly supplemented.

202. (E) Immune globulin is used for all these diagnoses.

203. (D) Lipase is the portion of pancreatic enzymes needed to calculate the dose for supplementation. There are various methods for determining the dose using lipase U/kg ingested fat or lipase U/kg body weight. Because dosing is based on lipase units, they should be equivalent when substituting products.

204. (E) Pain relief and inflammation are the primary concerns when treating a patient with an acute gout attack. Allopurinol decreases the production of uric acid and therefore should decrease future attacks, but it will not alleviate an acute attack.

205. (E) All these effects are recognized adverse events associated with theophylline use.

206. (D) Obesity and acute renal failure have both been associated with insulin resistance.

207. (E) All of these effects are recognized adverse events associated with oral iron therapy.

208. (B) Quinidine has a high incidence (up to 30%) of GI side effects. Nausea, vomiting, and diarrhea commonly occur initially. However, many patients develop tolerance to these side effects.

209. (B) Cellulose derivatives (e.g., Citrucel) and psyllium preparations (e.g., Metamucil) are bulk-forming laxatives. In addition to forming bulk, their absorption of water from the gut can alleviate watery diarrhea.

210. (E) Ergot alkaloids cause vasoconstriction. They should not be used in pregnant patients (due to decreased placental blood flow) or in any patient whose blood flow is compromised.

211. (E) Hepatotoxicity in the form of reversible cholestatic hepatitis has been associated with the estolate salt. It is most commonly seen in patients whose therapy has been longer than 10 days or who have had repeated courses.

212. (E) Anticholinergic agents may worsen the symptoms of all these conditions.

213. (A) Thrombocytopenia may occur in up to 25% of the patients receiving heparin.

214. (E) All of these drugs are known to interact with digoxin.

215. (E) All of these drugs may increase theophylline concentrations.

3

Microbiology and Public Health

DIRECTIONS (Questions 1–100): Each of the questions or incomplete statements below is followed by five suggested answers or completions. Select the **one answer** that is best in each case.

1. Rubella is another name for
    A. measles
    B. meningitis
    C. German measles
    D. scarlet fever
    E. mumps

2. Which of the following substances is used in combination with beta-lactam antibiotics to extend their spectrum of activity?
    A. Cilastatin
    B. Sulbactam
    C. Tazobactam
    D. Clavulanic acid
    E. All of the above

3. *Pasteurella pestis* is transmitted by
    A. rat flea
    B. dog bite
    C. vaccines

    D. fecal contamination of water
    E. food contamination

4. Mumps in children usually involves the
    A. salivary glands
    B. tonsils and throat
    C. sex glands
    D. pancreas and liver
    E. central nervous system

5. Gray patches on the tonsils or mucous membranes of the nose and throat are associated with
    A. measles
    B. mumps
    C. diphtheria
    D. German measles
    E. tetanus

6. Toxoids are
    A. obtained from culture filtrates of viable organisms
    B. bacterial vaccines
    C. nonspecific protein filtrates
    D. nonantigenic toxins
    E. unofficial toxins

7. The time of day when fevers tend to peak is
    A. 2 PM to 4 PM
    B. 4 AM to 6 AM
    C. 6 PM to 10 PM
    D. 10 AM to 12 PM
    E. 10 PM to 12 AM

8. In order to kill spores,
    A. autoclave for 15 to 20 minutes at 120 °C
    B. steam the medium for 15 to 20 minutes
    C. raise temperature slowly to 90 °C and maintain this temperature for 1 hour
    D. heat 15 to 30 minutes at 100 °C in moist heat on 3 successive days
    E. do A and B

9. Most food poisoning is caused by a species of
   A. typhus
   B. *Salmonella*
   C. *Shigella*
   D. tetanus
   E. *Pasteurella*

10. Agglutinins are
    A. antitoxins that lyse bacteria
    B. carbohydrates
    C. a product of bacterial secretions
    D. antibodies that cause bacteria to clump together
    E. nonspecific

11. Sterilization means
    A. freeing an object from life of any kind
    B. removal of organisms capable of causing infection
    C. inhibition of growth of bacteria
    D. removal of facultative anaerobes
    E. none of the above

12. Viruses and rickettsiae differ from bacteria in their food requirements because they
    A. can live only on synthetic media
    B. can multiply only in the presence of bacteria
    C. need sunlight for growth
    D. cannot survive without the presence of living tissue
    E. can grow only in soil

13. Thermal death point takes place when
    A. all bacteria of a given species are killed after 10 minutes of exposure
    B. all bacteria of a given species are killed after 20 minutes of exposure
    C. all bacteria are killed instantaneously
    D. half of the virulent organisms are killed
    E. lysis of bacteria begins

14. In young children, tetracyclines often cause
    A. agranulocytosis
    B. discoloration of teeth

C. conjunctivitis
D. muscular weakness
E. hyperplasia of the gums

15. Immunization against measles usually employs
    A. a measles toxoid
    B. gamma globulin
    C. a live attenuated virus
    D. live bacteria
    E. attenuated rickettsia

16. Which of the following antibiotics are effective in treating human cases of anthrax?
    A. Ciprofloxacin (oral or IV)
    B. Doxycycline (oral)
    C. Vancomycin (oral)
    D. A and B
    E. A, B, and C

17. An organ of the body that is often damaged permanently by rheumatic fever is the
    A. lung
    B. kidney
    C. heart
    D. liver
    E. spleen

18. Gas gangrene is commonly caused by
    A. *Pasteurella*
    B. *Clostridia*
    C. *Rickettsia*
    D. *Shigella*
    E. *Mycobacterium*

19. The mechanism of dry heat sterilization is primarily
    A. oxidation
    B. reduction
    C. coagulation
    D. denaturation
    E. none of the above

20. Bacteriophages are usually
   A. bacteria
   B. viruses
   C. lipoidal
   D. polysaccharides
   E. none of the above

21. An antibody is chemically
   A. a protein
   B. a polysaccharide
   C. an amino acid
   D. any foreign substance in the body
   E. none of the above

22. Scabies is a disease of the
   A. mouth
   B. skin
   C. liver
   D. lungs
   E. GI tract

23. Rocky Mountain spotted fever is caused by
   A. a virus
   B. a rickettsia
   C. a bacteria
   D. an amoeba
   E. none of the above

24. HEPA filters are widely used in
   A. autoclaves
   B. laminar flow hoods
   C. face masks
   D. oxygen masks
   E. gas sterilizers

25. A bacteriostatic agent has which of the following effects on bacteria?
   A. It kills bacteria on contact
   B. It enhances their growth
   C. It induces spore formation
   D. It inhibits multiplication of bacteria
   E. It dehydrates bacteria

26. An anaphylactic reaction is an indication
  A. that antibodies are not present in the blood
  B. of immunity
  C. of hypersensitivity to a given protein
  D. of the presence of typhoid bacilli
  E. of the infestation by trypanosomes

27. Although normally a harmless saprophyte, *Escherichia coli* is the most common source of
  A. peritonitis
  B. cholecystitis
  C. acute genitourinary infections
  D. pancreatitis
  E. appendicitis

28. In the United States, most cases of botulism can be traced to
  A. undercooked pork
  B. home-canned sausage and other meats
  C. home-canned vegetables and fruits
  D. fish from polluted water
  E. infected pastry

29. Vaccine prepared from a patient's own infection is called
  A. autogenous vaccine
  B. stock vaccine
  C. monovalent vaccine
  D. polyvalent vaccine
  E. simple vaccine

30. A common method to maintain the exponential phase of growth of microorganisms is
  A. heating
  B. repeated transfers
  C. super cooling
  D. adding electrolytes
  E. none of the above

31. Each of the following exert antimicrobial action by inhibiting cell wall synthesis **EXCEPT**
  A. cephalosporins
  B. penicillins
  C. bacitracin
  D. vancomycin
  E. novobiocin

32. "Disk tests" to determine sensitivity of microorganisms do not work well for polymyxins because
  A. the disks are unstable
  B. the large molecules diffuse poorly
  C. the zone of inhibition is too large
  D. polymyxins only work in vivo
  E. polymyxins have intense color

33. Which of the following drugs would be effective therapy for *Clostridium difficile* colitis or enterocolitis associated with *Staphylococcus aureus*?
  A. Vancomycin (IV)
  B. Vancomycin (oral)
  C. Doxycycline
  D. A and B
  E. A, B, and C

34. Which of the following reactions are considered type I hypersensitivity events?
  A. Anaphylaxis
  B. Allergic bronchospasm
  C. Immune thrombocytopenic purpura
  D. A and B
  E. A, B, and C

35. Furuncles and abscesses are most frequently caused by
  A. staphylococci
  B. streptococci
  C. gram-positive rods
  D. gram-negative rods
  E. spirochetes

36. Active infection gives little or no immunity to
  A. mumps
  B. gonorrhea
  C. smallpox
  D. measles
  E. chickenpox

37. After initial immunization with a series of tetanus toxoid, boosters should be given
  A. twice a year
  B. every 2 years
  C. every 4 years
  D. every 6 years
  E. every 10 years

38. The hepatitis B vaccine protects against infection with which of the following viruses?
  I. Hepatitis B
  II. Hepatitis D
  III. Hepatitis A

  A. I only
  B. II only
  C. III only
  D. I and II only
  E. II and III only

39. The causative organism of syphilis is
  A. *Vibrio comma*
  B. *Spirillum minor*
  C. *Borrelia refringens*
  D. *Treponema pallidum*
  E. none of the above

40. Rickettsial growth is enhanced by
  A. PABA
  B. sulfonamides
  C. chloromycetin
  D. tetracycline
  E. higher temperature

41. In which of the following are fungal infestations very resistant and difficult to eradicate?
   A. Ear
   B. Foot
   C. Scalp
   D. Nails
   E. Vaginal tract

42. An advantage of live virus vaccines over killed viral vaccines is
   A. better stability
   B. ease of titration
   C. longer immunity
   D. faster action
   E. none of the above

43. Rabies is readily carried by
   A. dogs
   B. bats
   C. cats
   D. A and B
   E. A, B, and C

44. Amebiasis is caused by a
   A. fungus
   B. bacteria
   C. protozoan parasite
   D. virus
   E. mold

45. Salmonellosis is usually transmitted by
   A. mosquitoes
   B. fleas
   C. animal bites
   D. contaminated food or drink
   E. bats

46. *Haemophilus influenzae* meningitis occurs in
   A. the elderly
   B. teenagers
   C. young children

    D. middle-aged adults
    E. all age groups

47. Rocky Mountain spotted fever is usually transmitted by
    A. mosquitoes
    B. flies
    C. fleas
    D. mountain lions
    E. ticks

48. A drug used as a preventative when traveling to areas in which malaria is endemic is
    A. human immune globulin
    B. chloroquine phosphate
    C. quinine
    D. malarial vaccine
    E. none of the above

49. Toxic shock syndrome is seen most commonly in
    A. elderly women
    B. sexually active males
    C. women of childbearing age
    D. postmenopausal females
    E. female homosexuals

50. Home-canned vegetables are frequently a cause of
    A. typhus
    B. botulism
    C. salmonellosis
    D. fever of unknown origin
    E. tetanus

51. Biting dogs or cats should be quarantined and observed for signs of rabies for
    A. 24 hours
    B. 48 hours
    C. 96 hours
    D. 7 to 10 days
    E. 3 weeks

52. Passive immunity to hepatitis A is conferred by
   A. hepatitis live vaccine
   B. *hepatitis toxoid*
   C. human immune globulin
   D. inactivated hepatitis A vaccine
   E. none of the above because it is not possible

53. The usual carrier for shistosomiasis is
   A. snails
   B. mosquitoes
   C. ticks
   D. warm-blooded animals
   E. lice

54. Which of the following agents are used to treat hepatitis C?
   A. lamvudine
   B. interferon
   C. interferon and ribavirin
   D. A and B
   E. A, B, and C

55. Hepatitis A is transmitted via which of the following routes?
   A. Fecal–oral
   B. Blood
   C. Aerosolization
   D. A and B
   E. A, B, and C

56. Which of the following antibiotics or group of antibiotics does **NOT** act by inhibition of cell membrane function?
   A. Erythromycins
   B. Amphotericin B
   C. Colistin
   D. Nystatin
   E. Polymyxins

57. Cross-resistance to antibiotics is most closely related to
   A. method of production
   B. chemical structure
   C. genetic factors
   D. racial origin
   E. individual resistance

58. Which of the following are gram-negative bacilli?
   A. *N gonorrhoeae*
   B. *N meningitiditis*
   C. *Clostridium difficile*
   D. *Klebsiella pneumoniae*
   E. All of the above

59. Isoniazid is very active against
   A. streptococci
   B. staphylococci
   C. mycobacteria
   D. vibrio
   E. resistant staphylococci

60. Miconazole is particularly effective against
   A. vaginal candidiasis
   B. tricophyton infestations
   C. coccidiomycosis
   D. blastomycosis
   E. histoplasmosis

61. Hemolysins exert a marked effect on
   A. lymphocytes
   B. white blood cells
   C. red blood cells
   D. clotting
   E. bone marrow

62. Streptococcal infections are commonly a cause of secondary
   A. reinfection
   B. cardiac arrest
   C. undulant fever
   D. rheumatic fever
   E. sleeping sickness

63. Which of the following is the drug recommended for the treatment of chlamydial infections in adolescents and adults?
   A. Doxycycline
   B. Azithromycin
   C. Ofloxacin
   D. Erythromycin base
   E. None of the above

64. Which of the following statements is (are) true regarding varicella-zoster virus (VZV) (chickenpox) infections?

  I. Average incubation period may range from 10 to 21 days

  II. Contagiousness of infected persons begins approximately 1 to 2 days before the onset of rash and ends when all lesions are crusted

  III. It is transmitted via direct contact, droplet, or aerosol of vesicular fluid of skin lesions

  A. I only
  B. III only
  C. I and II only
  D. II and III only
  E. I, II, and III

65. Which of the following drug(s) is (are) recommended by the American Heart Association as a prophylactic regimen(s) prior to dental surgery in patients who are at risk of bacterial endocarditis?

  I. Erythromycin
  II. Amoxicillin
  III. Azithromycin

  A. I only
  B. III only
  C. I and II only
  D. II and III only
  E. I, II, and III

66. Candidates for the hepatitis A vaccine include
  A. persons living in areas of endemic hepatitis A outbreaks
  B. military personnel
  C. child-care center employees
  D. users of illicit injectable drugs
  E. all of the above

67. The drug of choice for vaginal trichomoniasis in a nonpregnant woman is
  A. norfloxacin
  B. co-trimoxazole
  C. metronidazole

D. amoxicillin
E. none of the above

68. Which of the following statements regarding attenuated viruses is (are) true?
    A. Contain altered, weakened, or avirulent bacteria or virus
    B. May be dangerous in an immunocompromised person
    C. Induce active immunity
    D. Are usually more immunogenic than killed vaccines
    E. All of the above

69. Which of the following vaccines is (are) recommended by the American Academy of Immunization Practices as part of the routine immunization series for children from birth to 12 years?
    A. Hepatitis B vaccine
    B. *Haemophilus influenzae* type B
    C. Varicella virus vaccine
    D. Measles, mumps, rubella (MMR) vaccine
    E. All of the above

70. Which of the following statements is (are) true regarding post-varicella (chickenpox) infections?
    I. VZV becomes latent in sensory nerve ganglia without clinical manifestation
    II. Latent virus reactivation causes herpes zoster
    III. Approximately 85% of the population will experience herpes zoster during an average lifespan

    A. I only
    B. III only
    C. I and II only
    D. II and III only
    E. I, II, and III

71. Oral acyclovir is used to treat
    A. varicella (chickenpox)
    B. shingles
    C. initial episodes of genital herpes
    D. recurrent episodes of genital herpes
    E. all of the above

72. The prevention of gonococcal ophthalmia neonatorum is required by law in most states. Which of the following drugs is (are) recommended as a prophylactic agent(s) and should be administered to all newborn infants?
   A. Silver nitrate (1%) aqueous solution
   B. Erythromycin (0.5%) ophthalmic ointment
   C. Idoxuridine (0.1%) solution
   D. Vidarabine (3%) ointment
   E. A and B

73. Which of the following drugs is (are) recommended as single-dose regimens administered with oral doxycycline or azithromycin for the treatment of uncomplicated gonococcal infections?
   I.   Ceftriaxone 125 mg (IM)
   II. Ciprofloxacin 500 mg (PO)
   III. Cefixime 400 mg (PO)

   A. I only
   B. III only
   C. I and II only
   D. II and III only
   E. I, II, and III

74. Primary or secondary syphilis in adults should be treated with a single dose of
   A. benzathine penicillin G, 2.4 million units IM
   B. ciprofloxacin 500 mg PO
   C. acyclovir 800 mg PO
   D. A and B
   E. none of the above

75. Which of the following organisms are gram-negative cocci?
   A. *Neisseria gonorrhoeae*
   B. *Bacteroides fragilis*
   C. *Klebsiella pneumoniae*
   D. *Escherichia coli*
   E. All of the above

76. Which of the following statement(s) regarding varicella virus vaccine is (are) true?
    I. It is recommended for postexposure prophylaxis of varicella
    II. It is a dead virus vaccine
    III. The seroconversion rate is greater than 90% after the administration of one dose to children aged 12 months to 12 years

    A. I only
    B. III only
    C. I and II only
    D. II and III only
    E. I, II, and III

77. Which of the following organisms are gram-positive cocci?
    I. *Staphylococcus aureus*
    II. *Streptococcus pneumoniae*
    III. *Clostridium difficile*

    A. I only
    B. III only
    C. I and II only
    D. II and III only
    E. I, II, and III

78. Which of the following laboratory values is associated with an infection?
    A. Increased WBCs with a "shift to the left"
    B. Positive Gram stain
    C. Increased blood urea nitrogen
    D. A and B
    E. A, B, and C

79. Which of the following statements regarding minimal inhibitory concentration (MIC) is (are) true?

   I. MIC is the lowest antibiotic concentration that inhibits visible bacterial growth

   II. MICs are used to determine bacterial susceptibility to a particular antimicrobial

  III. MIC ≤ MBC (minimum bactericidal concentration)

   A. I only
   B. III only
   C. I and II only
   D. II and III only
   E. I, II, and III

80. Which of the following screening tests is (are) used to test antibodies to the human immunodeficiency virus (HIV)?

   A. Enzyme-linked immunosorbent assay (ELISA)
   B. Western blot
   C. Cold hemagglutinin
   D. A and B
   E. A, B, and C

81. Lyme disease is caused by which of the following organisms?

   A. *Shigella* sp
   B. *Enterobacter aerogenes*
   C. *Borrelia burgdorferi*
   D. *Listeria monocytogenes*
   E. None of the above

82. Which of the following statements regarding passive immunity is (are) true?

   I. Develops in response to an infection

   II. Provides life-long immunity

  III. Protects almost immediately

   A. I only
   B. III only
   C. I and II only
   D. II and III only
   E. I, II, and III

83. Which of the following agents is used to treat Lyme disease?
  A. Amoxicillin
  B. Metronidazole
  C. Amphotericin
  D. Ceftriaxone
  E. None of the above

84. Initial empiric treatment of tuberculosis in an adult should include which of the following drugs?
  A. Isoniazid
  B. Rifampin
  C. Pyrazinamide
  D. Ethambutol
  E. All of the above

85. Which of the following groups are **NOT** candidates for lindane therapy?
  A. Pregnant and lactating women
  B. Children under 2 years of age
  C. Persons with extensive dermatitis
  D. A and B
  E. A, B, and C

86. A positive reaction to a tuberculin skin (PPD) test indicates which of the following?
  A. Presence of active disease
  B. Implies past or present infection with tuberculosis
  C. Immunity to invasion by tubercle bacillus
  D. Susceptible to invasion by tubercle bacillus
  E. None of the above

87. Which of the following are examples of type I immediate or allergic hypersensitivity?
  A. Hay fever
  B. Pollen allergy
  C. Insect venom hypersensitivity
  D. Allergic asthma
  E. All of the above

88. Which of the following is considered a type IV or delayed hypersensitivity reaction?
    A. Eczema
    B. Food allergy
    C. Drug hypersensitivity
    D. Tuberculin skin test reactions
    E. None of the above

89. Which of the following is the most prevalent immune globulin in the body?
    A. IgG
    B. IgA
    C. IgM
    D. IgE
    E. IgD

90. Which of the following is (are) advantages of the Salk polio vaccine when compared to the Sabin polio vaccine?
    I. Inactivated virus vaccine eliminates the risk of causing polio
    II. Easier route of administration
    III. Greater efficacy

    A. I only
    B. III only
    C. I and II only
    D. II and III only
    E. I, II, and III

91. Lyme disease is transmitted to humans via
    A. cats
    B. deer ticks
    C. spiders
    D. guinea pigs
    E. none of the above

92. Postexposure prophylaxis for rabies after a bite from a suspected rabid domestic dog or cat would include
    I. rabies immune globulin (RIG)
    II. rabies vaccine
    III. tetanus toxoid

A. I only
B. III only
C. I and II only
D. II and III only
E. I, II, and III

93. Which of the following forms should be completed to report an adverse reaction to a vaccine?
   I. Vaccine Adverse Event Reporting System
   II. FDA MedWatch
   III. USP Product Problem Report

   A. I only
   B. III only
   C. I and II only
   D. II and III only
   E. I, II, and III

94. Which of the following vaccines is contraindicated in breast-feeding women?
   A. Attenuated virus
   B. Killed virus
   C. Live virus
   D. Attenuated bacteria
   E. None of the above

95. Which of the following is (are) live viral vaccines?
   I. Oral polio vaccine
   II. Oral typhoid vaccine
   III. Influenza vaccines

   A. I only
   B. III only
   C. I and II only
   D. II and III only
   E. I, II, and III

96. Which of the following drugs is (are) used in prophylactic regimens for malaria?
  I. Mefloquine
  II. Primaquine
  III. Pyrimethamine–sulfadoxine

  A. I only
  B. III only
  C. I and II only
  D. II and III only
  E. I, II, and III

97. Which of the following immunologics is (are) used as treatment rather than immunization or detection?
  I. Antivenins
  II. Interferons
  III. Anergy tests

  A. I only
  B. III only
  C. I and II only
  D. II and III only
  E. I, II, and III

98. Which of the following statements regarding the inactivated trivalent influenza virus vaccine is **TRUE**?
  A. Each year the vaccine virus strains remain the same as the previous year
  B. Persons with known hypersensitivity to eggs are candidates for the vaccine
  C. All inactivated influenza vaccines are split virus preparations
  D. Vaccination is advised for persons infected with HIV
  E. All of the above

99. Which of the following groups is (are) candidates for influenza virus vaccination?
  A. Persons greater than 65 years old
  B. Nursing home residents
  C. Adults with chronic pulmonary problems

D. Children with asthma

E. All of the above

100. Which of the following contraceptive methods is (are) associated with the lowest pregnancy rate?

A. Vasectomy

B. Tubal ligation

C. Periodic abstinence

D. Condom with spermicide

E. Spermicide alone

Microbiology and Public Health

Answers and Discussion

1. **(C)** The common name is German measles.

2. **(E)** All these substances are used to extend spectrums. Specific combinations include imipenem/cilastatin, piperacillin/tazobactam, ampicillin/sulbactam, and amoxicillin/clavulanic acid.

3. **(A)** The rat flea is the usual carrier.

4. **(A)** Mumps seldom involves the throat or tonsils in children.

5. **(C)** The gray patches are due to the formation of a pseudomembrane.

6. **(A)** Exotoxins are treated with formaldehyde and then purified.

7. **(C)** Fever is lower in the morning and tends to peak in late afternoon or early evening.

8. **(D)** The methods listed in A, B, and C will not kill most spores.

9. (B) *Salmonella typhimurium* is the most common of the salmonellae causing this.

10. (D) Agglutination means clumping or aggregation.

11. (A) Sterilization is an absolute term.

12. (D) Viruses and rickettsiae require living tissue, but bacteria will grow on synthetic media.

13. (A) It is the temperature at which this occurs.

14. (B) This is an irreversible discoloration that occurs during the tooth-forming years.

15. (C) Rubella and measles vaccinations employ a live attenuated virus.

16. (D) *Bacillus anthracis,* a gram-positive bacillus, is the causative agent of anthrax. Spores of this bacterium are used in germ warfare. Prophylaxis and treatment may be effective with ciprofloxacin 500 mg twice daily or doxycycline 100 mg twice daily. Vancomycin suffers from poor absorption properties when administered orally and is only indicated for treatment of pseudomembranous colitis or enterocolitis associated with *Staphylococcus aureus*; it is not effective in other types of infection.

17. (C) Rheumatic fever may cause weakening of the valves.

18. (B) The toxin produced by *Clostridia* spreads rapidly and has a necrotizing action.

19. (A) Oxidation speeds up the process markedly.

20. (B) Bacteriophages are highly specific viruses that use bacteria as hosts.

21. (A) Antibodies are proteins formed in response to antigens.

22. (B) It is a common type of dermatitis.

23. (B) Most of the spotted fevers are rickettsial in origin.

24. (B) These are filters that remove particles from air.

25. (D) Bacteriostatics inhibit the growth phase.

26. (C) A massive amount of histamine is produced by a foreign protein or antigen.

27. (C) Infection usually occurs only under a specialized set of conditions that promote overgrowth.

28. (C) Botulism is caused by improper handling (usually poor sealing) or storage.

29. (A) Autogenous means self-generated.

30. (B) Repeated transfers prevent exhaustion of the medium and prevent buildup of toxic metabolic products.

31. (E) Novobiocin acts by inhibiting nucleic acid synthesis.

32. (B) Poor diffusion in agar makes the zone of inhibition very small.

33. (B) Parenteral administration of vancomycin *does not* achieve therapeutically effective fecal levels and should not be used to treat *C difficile* colitis or enterocolitis associated with *S aureus*. Oral vancomycin is only indicated for treatment of pseudomembranous colitis or enterocolitis associated with *S aureus*; it is not effective in other types of infection.

34. (D) A type I hypersensitivity reaction is primarily mediated by immunoglobulins E and G with an immediate onset (often within 15 minutes). Typical reactions include insect venom hypersensitivity, anaphylaxis, allergic bronchospasm, and urticaria. Type II reactions are primarily mediated by IgG, IgM, and complement, and include reactions such as Graves' disease, immune thrombocytopenic purpura, hemolytic anemia, and Goodpasture's syndrome.

35. **(A)** Furuncles and abscesses are prototypical staph lesions.

36. **(B)** Repeated infections and relapses are the rule in gonococcal infections. Antibodies are quite strain-specific or have little protective ability. The others give lasting immunity.

37. **(E)** Routine booster doses are recommended every 10 years.

38. **(D)** Protection against hepatitis A infection is conferred by the hepatitis A vaccine. Because hepatitis D virus can only infect and cause illness in people infected with hepatitis B and because hepatitis D virus requires a coat of hepatitis B surface antigens to become infective, hepatitis B vaccines confer protection against both B and D virus infection.

39. **(D)** Only *T pallidum* causes syphilis, but the spirochete *B refringens* is often confused with *T pallidum.*

40. **(B)** All but sulfonamides inhibit growth. Sulfonamides are contraindicated.

41. **(D)** Nail infections require months of treatment and sometimes surgical removal of the nails. The other types respond quickly to the appropriate antifungal agents.

42. **(C)** Killed virus vaccines provide only short-term immunity, whereas "live" vaccines give longer term immunity. There is little difference in stability, ease of titer, or onset of action.

43. **(E)** Rabies has a wide host range that includes all warm-blooded animals.

44. **(C)** Amebiasis is caused by the protozoan parasite *Entamoeba histolytica.*

45. (D) The introduction of *Salmonella* is usually by ingestion of contaminated food or drink. Human carriers should not work as food handlers.

46. (C) *Haemophilus influenzae* meningitis occurs primarily in children under 6 years of age.

47. (E) The disease is almost always transmitted by wood or dog ticks.

48. (B) Only chloroquine is recommended. Quinine may be useful in only a few cases. Chloroquinine should be taken beginning 2 weeks before arrival and for 4 weeks after leaving the endemic area.

49. (C) Most (90% or more) of the cases are in women of childbearing age. Most cases occur in women using tampons.

50. (B) *C botulinum* is found in soil. It can contaminate vegetables that are not washed well and cooked properly.

51. (D) Symptoms of rabies should appear in dogs or cats within 7 to 10 days.

52. (C) Human immune globulin confers short-term passive immunity. No toxoid is ever used, and live or inactivated vaccines do not confer passive-type immunity.

53. (A) Part of the life-cycle of schistosomes is in snails.

54. (E) All these agents have been used with some efficacy to treat acute and chronic hepatitis C infections. Interferon has had almost complete success in reversing acute hepatitis C when started shortly after exposure. Success rates are low for all drugs in the treatment of chronic hepatitis C.

55. (A) Hepatitis A is transmitted person to person via the fecal–oral route. The infectious agent is found in the feces at peak concentrations 1 to 2 weeks before the onset of symptoms. Common sources of outbreaks may be related to contaminated food or water. Hepatitis B is infectious via blood, serum-derived fluids, saliva, semen, and vaginal fluids. The most common modes of transmission include needle-stick accidents, contaminated intravenous drug use, perinatal exposure, and sexual exposure.

56. **(A)** All but erythromycins act by inhibiting all membrane function. Cephalosporins act through inhibition of protein synthesis.

57. **(B)** Antibiotics of similar chemical structure usually have the same mechanism of action and cross-resistance is common.

58. **(D)** *K pneumoniae* are gram-negative bacilli. *N Gonorrhoeae* and *N meningitiditis* are gram-negative cocci. *C difficile* are gram-positive bacilli.

59. **(C)** Isoniazid has little activity against all but mycobacteria. It is particularly effective against *Mycobacterium tuberculosis*.

60. **(A)** Miconazole is more effective topically and is too toxic when given for systemic fungal infections. It is almost ineffective against tricophyton.

61. **(C)** Hemolysins disrupt red blood cells by lysis, but have little effect on other blood cells or blood-forming organs.

62. **(D)** Rheumatic fever is almost always a secondary effect following some streptococcal infections, particularly in children.

63. **(E)** All of these drugs are effective regimens for the treatment of chlamydia. The Centers for Disease Control and Prevention (CDC) recommended regimens include doxycycline or azithromycin. Safety and efficacy of azithromycin in patients under 15 years of age have not been established. Additional alternatives are erythromycin or ofloxacin.

64. **(E)** Chickenpox, a highly contagious disease caused by VZV, is transmitted via direct contact, droplet or aerosol of

vesicular fluid of skin lesions, or by secretions from the respiratory tract. Average incubation period is 14 to 16 days, but can be as long as 10 to 21 days. Full body lesion crusting usually occurs 4 to 5 days after rash onset.

65. (C) Amoxicillin (2 g PO 1 hour before procedure) is the standard prophylactic regimen for dental surgery. In patients who are penicillin/amoxicillin allergic, cephalexin, azithromycin or erythromycin and clindamycin are recommended alternatives by the American Heart Association guidelines published in 1997. (See *JAMA* 277:1794, 1997.)

66. (E) All of the mentioned groups are candidates for preexposure prophylaxis hepatitis A vaccination.

67. (C) Trichomoniasis, caused by the protozoan *Trichomonas vaginalis,* typically causes a malodorous, yellow-green discharge with vulvar irritation in women. The CDC–recommended regimen is metronidazole 2 g PO in a single dose or 500 mg BID for 7 days.

68. (E) All of these statements are true. Live vaccines may be dangerous in immunocompromised patients because they may not be capable of mounting an effective defense against even avirulent bacteria/viruses. Attenuated viruses often produce serum antibody for longer durations.

69. (E) All of these vaccines are recommended in routine immunization series.

70. (C) VZV remains latent in the ganglia until reactivation as herpes zoster infection, which develops most frequently among immunocompromised persons and the elderly. Only 15% of the population will develop herpes zoster infections.

71. (E) Acyclovir, an antiviral, has inhibitory in vitro activity against herpes simplex virus 1 and 2, VZV, Epstein–Barr virus (EBV), and cytomegalovirus (CMV). This drug is used for the acute treatment of herpes zoster (shingles), varicella (chickenpox), and initial and recurrent episodes of genital herpes.

72. (E) Silver nitrate (1%) aqueous solution, erythromycin (0.5%) ointment, or tetracycline (1%) ophthalmic ointment in a single application are recommended regimens for ophthalmia neonatorum prophylaxis. Idoxuridine and vidarabine are not effective as they possess only antiviral activity.

73. (E) Any one of these regimens is recommended therapy by the CDC. Concomitant therapy with doxycycline or azithromycin is also used because coinfection with *C trachomatis* is common.

74. (A) Parenteral penicillin G is effective in achieving local cure and preventing later complications in most individuals with primary or secondary syphilis and is recommended by the CDC. For patients allergic to penicillin, 2 weeks of oral doxycycline or tetracycline is recommended.

75. (A) *Neisseria gonorrhoeae* are gram-negative cocci. All other organisms are gram-negative bacilli.

76. (B) VZV is a live attenuated virus vaccine recommended for routine immunization in children aged 12 months to 12 years and in adults who have not contracted varicella previously. This vaccine is not recommended for postexposure prophylaxis. Varicella zoster immune globulin (VZIG), if administered within 72 hours of exposure, prevents clinical varicella in the majority of susceptible healthy children. Seroconversion rates with one dose of the varicella vaccine in children over 12 years of age is over 90% at 4 years postvaccination.

77. (C) *Streptococcus pneumoniae* and *Staphylococcus aureus* are gram-positive cocci. *Clostridium difficile* is a gram-positive bacilli organism.

78. (D) An increase in WBCs with a rise in immature forms or bands (left shift) is a common laboratory result that indicates an infection. A positive Gram stain can indicate the presence, quantity, and type of bacteria. Blood urea nitrogen is typically unaffected by infectious processes unless renal dysfunction is also present.

79. (E) MIC is the lowest antibiotic concentration (or highest dilution) that inhibits visible bacterial growth and is commonly used to determine bacterial susceptibility or resistance to a particular antimicrobial agent. MBC is the lowest antibiotic concentration that kills 99.9% of the bacteria.

80. (D) ELISA is the most common screening test used to detect HIV in donated blood as it is inexpensive and reliable. The Western blot detects HIV antibodies to specific HIV proteins and glycoproteins. Cold hemagglutinin is an antibody that reacts to antigen on red blood cells and is used in diagnosing *Mycoplasma pneumoniae.*

81. (C) *Borrelia burgdorferi,* a spirochete, is the cause of Lyme disease. Histologic staining is often difficult because affected tissues may not contain a large number of spirochetes and the organism is not grown easily in the laboratory.

82. (B) Active immunity develops after infection or via administration of a vaccine or toxoid, usually requires several weeks to induce, and provides long-lasting immunity (several years). In contrast, passive immunity develops after the administration of an immunoglobulin or transferred from another living host (during pregnancy) and provides protection immediately but is of short duration (usually only days or weeks).

83. (D) Ceftriaxone is commonly used to treat Lyme disease.

84. (E) The CDC recommends that a four drug regimen with isoniazid, rifampin, pyrazinamide, and streptomycin or ethambutol is preferred initial and empiric treatment for tuberculosis in children and adults.

85. (E) Lindane, an ectoparasiticide, is used to treat lice infestations and scabies. Although lindane has a Food and Drug Administration pregnancy rating B, the CDC does not recommend its use in pregnant or lactating women. Significant systemic absorption may occur resulting in CNS toxicity, including seizures. Toxic effects are more likely in infants and children under 2 and in individuals with extensive dermatitis.

86. **(B)** A positive tuberculin reaction does not necessarily indicate the presence of active disease but implies a past or present infection. Further diagnostic tests (i.e., chest x-ray, microbiologic exam of sputum) are required before a diagnosis of tuberculosis can be validated.

87. **(E)** Immediate/allergic hypersensitivity usually occurs within 15 minutes and is primarily mediated by immunoglobulins E and G, basophils, or mast cells. All of the examples provided may be classified as type I responses.

88. **(D)** Delayed hypersensitivity reactions are cell-mediated immune responses, mediated primarily by T-lymphocytes and usually occurring after 24 to 72 hours. Drug and food allergies and eczema are examples of immediate hypersensitivity reactions.

89. **(A)** IgG is the most abundant of the immunoglobulins in the human body, found in typical serum concentrations of 8 to 16 mg/mL. Decreasing concentrations in the human body are IgA, IgM, IgD, and IgE. IgE levels are often elevated in allergic or parasitic reactions.

90. **(A)** The inactivated polio virus vaccine (Salk) eliminates the risk of inducing polio and therefore is preferred for immunization of adults, because they are more likely to incur oral polio vaccine poliomyelitis than are children. The Salk vaccine is administered subcutaneously. Both vaccines provide similar efficacy (95% to 100%).

91. **(B)** Deer ticks carry *Borrelia burgdorferi,* the spirochete responsible for causing Lyme disease.

92. **(C)** Rabies immune globulin and rabies vaccine are indicated prophylaxis for bites from rabid or suspected rabid domestic cats or dogs.

93. **(A)** A Vaccine Adverse Event Reporting System report should be completed when an adverse event has occurred following the administration of a vaccine. An FDA MedWatch form is usually indicated for adverse events or product problems associated with drugs or devices. The USP

Product Problem Reporting Program is designed to collect data regarding product defects and problems.

94. (E) Neither killed nor live vaccines affect the safety of breast-feeding for mothers or infants. Breast-feeding does not affect immunization adversely.

95. (A) Oral polio vaccine is a live virus vaccine. Both typhoid and influenza vaccines are bacterial vaccines.

96. (C) Mefloquine and primaquine are typically used in prophylactic regimens. Pyrimethamine–sulfadoxine is indicated only for treatment of malaria.

97. (C) Antivenins are used to treat certain insect or snake bites. Interferons are used to treat various viral infections. Anergy tests are used to diagnose specific sensitivity reactions.

98. (D) For persons infected with HIV, vaccination is recommended because influenza infection may result in serious illness and complications. The effectiveness of the vaccine may be reduced due to inability of HIV patients to mount an antibody response. Despite this deficiency, administration in this population is still recommended. Each year the types of virus strains are selected on previous years' infections and anticipated changes or trends. Persons with known hypersensitivity to eggs should not be administered the influenza vaccine. The inactivated influenza vaccine is available as both split-virus and whole virus preparations.

99. (E) All these groups are at increased risk of influenza-related complications and should receive annual influenza vaccinations.

100. (A) The following pregnancy rates are approximates: vasectomy (0.15%); tubal ligation (0.40%); periodic abstinence (20.00%); condom with spermicide (4.00% to 6.00%); spermicide alone (21.00%).

4

Chemistry and Biochemistry

DIRECTIONS (Questions 1–140): Each of the questions or incomplete statements below is followed by five suggested answers or completions. Select the **one answer** that is best in each case.

1. Which of the following diuretics do **NOT** cause potassium loss?
   A. Furosemide
   B. Chlorthalidone
   C. Triamterene
   D. Hydrochlorothiazide
   E. Metolazone

2. Sodium polysterene sulfonate (Kayexalate) is a cation ion exchange resin that is used clinically to decrease the level of
   A. aluminum
   B. potassium
   C. magnesium
   D. calcium
   E. chloride

3. The principal hydrolysis degradation product of aspirin is
   A. salicylic acid
   B. methyl salicylate
   C. salicylamide
   D. acrolein
   E. acetyl chloride

4. Grignard reagents usually contain
   A. Co
   B. Cu
   C. Fe
   D. Pb
   E. Mg

5. Nuclear magnetic resonance (NMR) is used mainly for
   A. quantitative assays
   B. irradiation
   C. identification of chemical substances
   D. radioisotopes
   E. none of the above

6. How many molecules of NaOH will react with 6.06×10^{23} molecules of sulfuric acid?
   A. 6.06×10^{23}
   B. 12.12×10^{23}
   C. 3.03×10^{23}
   D. 6.06×10^{46}
   E. $6.06 \times 10^{11.5}$

7. Which of the following calcium salts has the highest percentage of elemental calcium?
   A. Carbonate
   B. Citrate
   C. Glubionate
   D. Gluconate
   E. Lactate

8. Which of the following drugs can increase potassium levels?
   A. Corticosteroids
   B. Amphotericin B
   C. ACE inhibitors
   D. Furosemide
   E. Hydrochlorothiazide

9. Adsorption is a (an)
   A. irreversible chemical reaction
   B. reversible chemical reaction

C. complexation phenomenon
D. light-induced reaction
E. physical phenomenon

10. Fluorinated hydrocarbons are often used as
    A. general anesthetics
    B. hypnotics
    C. antiarrhythmics
    D. antihypertensives
    E. diuretics

11. Protein hydrolysates consist mainly of
    A. enzymes
    B. enzyme acids
    C. nitrites
    D. amino acids
    E. nitrates

12. All of the following statement about Technetium-99 are true EXCEPT that
    A. it is commonly used for imaging in medicine
    B. its half-life is 6 hours
    C. it emits gamma rays
    D. it can be compounded in a non-radiopharmaceutical area
    E. it is produced from molybdenum

13. A normal solution contains
    A. 1 g equivalent weight of solute in 1000 g of solution
    B. 1 g equivalent weight of solute in 1000 cc of solvent
    C. 1 g equivalent weight of solute in 1000 cc of solution
    D. 1 g molecular weight of solute in 1000 cc of solvent
    E. 1 g molecular weight of solute in 1000 cc of solution

14. In preparations used for gastric distress, aluminum hydroxide combines antacid action with
    A. laxative action
    B. coating action
    C. diuretic action
    D. histamine antagonist action
    E. preservative action

15. The principal oxidation product of ethylene glycol is
A. ethanol
B. citric acid
C. carbon monoxide
D. oxalic acid
E. acetaldehyde

16. What type of disease is suspected when an antinuclear antibody (ANA) test is ordered?
A. Rheumatic disease
B. Cardiac disease
C. Hepatic disease
D. Renal disease
E. Neurologic disorder

17. Oxidation of which alcohols yield ketones?
A. All
B. Primary
C. Secondary
D. Tertiary
E. Quarternary

18. Functional groups on organic molecules determine
A. solubility
B. reactivity
C. in vivo stability
D. A and B
E. A, B, and C

19. A general formula for an aldehyde is
A. ROH
B. RCHO
C. RCOOH
D. R—O—R
E. none of the above

20. Cellulose is a polysaccharide found in
A. plants
B. soil
C. human cells

D. animal fat
E. animal protein

21. Dimercaprol (BAL) acts as an antidote by a process called
    A. oxidation
    B. reduction
    C. chelation
    D. absorption
    E. adsorption

22. An ion that often shows expectorant action is
    A. iodide
    B. phosphate
    C. fluoride
    D. iodate
    E. perchlorate

23. Radioactive strontium is used as a
    A. diagnostic for thyroid function
    B. diagnostic bone scan
    C. medium for kidney imaging
    D. suppressant for blood dyscrasias
    E. suppressant for aplastic anemia

24. In the treatment of Wilson's disease, penicillamine is used to promote the excretion of
    A. copper
    B. calcium
    C. magnesium
    D. chromium
    E. manganese

25. Purified water is usually rendered sterile and pyrogen-free by
    A. repeated distillation
    B. gas sterilization
    C. autoclaving
    D. filtration
    E. freeze drying

26. Sorbic acid is used as a (an)
   A. antioxidant
   B. suspending agent
   C. mold and yeast inhibitor
   D. disintegrator
   E. filler

27. Chlorides may be precipitated from solution by the reagent
   A. potassium hydroxide
   B. silver nitrate
   C. lithium bromide
   D. sodium thiosulfate
   E. sodium metabisulfite

28. Which of the following is **NOT** classified as an inert gas?
   A. Nitrogen
   B. Helium
   C. Neon
   D. Argon
   E. Radon

29. Which of the following salts is used to treat contact dermatitis?
   A. Titanium
   B. Arsenic
   C. Tin
   D. Antimony
   E. Zirconium

30. Which of the following products is not considered an antioxidant?
   A. Vitamin C
   B. Vitamin E
   C. Beta-carotene
   D. Vitamin K
   E. Vitamin A

31. Which of the following IV medications should be filtered during administration?
   A. Amphotericin B
   B. Nitroglycerin
   C. Insulin

D. Mannitol
E. Lipid emulsion

32. The least stable of the water-soluble vitamins is
  A. ascorbic acid
  B. cyanocobalamin
  C. thiamine
  D. folic acid
  E. niacin

33. Which is **NOT** an essential amino acid?
  A. Threonine
  B. Tryptophane
  C. Valine
  D. Glutamine
  E. Methionine

34. A substance found commonly in fermented foods that can be toxic when monoamine oxidase (MAO) inhibitors are used is
  A. ADP
  B. STP
  C. tyramine
  D. histidine
  E. phenylalanine

35. Sodium nitroprusside is metabolized to which of the following compounds?
  A. Thiocyanate (cyanide)
  B. Copper
  C. Nitroglycerin
  D. Depo-prusside
  E. Nadolol

36. Which substance yields the largest number of calories per gram?
  A. Carbohydrates
  B. Proteins
  C. Minerals
  D. Fats
  E. Vitamins

37. The active proteolytic enzyme in gastric juice is
   A. pepsinogen
   B. pepsin
   C. bilirubin
   D. trypsin
   E. secretin

38. A normal value for fasting glucose in blood is
   A. 110 mg/dL
   B. 140 mg/dL
   C. 150 mg/dL
   D. 180 mg/dL
   E. 195 mg/dL

39. Which of the following decreases the effect of warfarin?
   A. Insulin
   B. Cimetidine
   C. Metronidazole
   D. Phenobarbital
   E. Ephedrine

40. Which of the following is a polysaccharide?
   A. Saccharin
   B. Starch
   C. Lactose
   D. Sodium cyclamine
   E. Maltose

41. The main carbohydrate of the blood is
   A. D-fructose
   B. mannitol
   C. D-glucose
   D. sorbitose
   E. L-glucose

42. A deficiency of which of the following vitamins can cause night blindness?
   A. D
   B. K
   C. A
   D. E
   E. B complex

43. Which of the following is present in all connective tissue?
   A. Mucoids
   B. Lipids
   C. Albuminoid
   D. All of the above
   E. None of the above

44. Vitamin K is necessary for
   A. prevention of rickets
   B. prevention of pernicious anemia
   C. formation of prothrombin
   D. formation of DNA
   E. muscle tone

45. Which of the following furnishes the most energy to muscles?
   A. ACTH
   B. LSD
   C. RNA
   D. DNA
   E. ATP

46. Follicle-stimulating hormone and interstitial cell-stimulating hormone are produced by the
   A. islets of Langerhans
   B. thymus gland
   C. thyroid gland
   D. pineal gland
   E. pituitary gland

47. Which of the following statements about insulin is (are) TRUE?
   A. Insulin is a hormone
   B. Insulin is a protein
   C. Insulin is secreted by the islets of Langerhans
   D. Insulin is rapidly distributed throughout extracellular fluid
   E. All of the above

48. The average life span of a red blood cell is about
   A. 7 days
   B. 14 days
   C. 3 weeks
   D. 1–2 months
   E. 4 months

49. The protein precursor of thyroxin is
   A. ornithine
   B. threonine
   C. tryptophan
   D. thyroglobulin
   E. thyroxinogen

50. The fat-soluble vitamins are
   A. B complex, C, and D
   B. A, D, E, and K
   C. A, B, C, and D
   D. B complex, E, and K
   E. A, B complex, and D

51. Each molecule of vitamin B_{12} contains an atom of
   A. potassium
   B. sodium
   C. cobalt
   D. calcium
   E. zinc

52. Zinc is most important for
   A. blood cell formation
   B. bone formation
   C. oxidative processes
   D. normal growth
   E. muscle contractions

53. Death due to cyanide poisoning results from
   A. cyanide–hemoglobin complex formation
   B. cyanide combining with red blood cells
   C. cyanide inhibiting cytochrome oxidase
   D. coronary vessel occlusion
   E. none of the above

54. Elevation of blood uric acid levels tends to produce
   A. dizziness
   B. dyspnea
   C. hypertension
   D. muscular weakness
   E. gout

55. Which of the following stimulates hepatic microsomal enzymes?
   A. Phenacemide
   B. Mannitol
   C. Phenobarbital
   D. Urea
   E. ASA

56. The nucleic acids, RNA and DNA, play important roles in the biosynthesis of protein. A sugar inherent in their structure is
   A. glucose
   B. sucrose
   C. fructose
   D. sorbose
   E. none of the above

57. Although the prostaglandins are hormone-like, they more closely resemble which of the following chemically?
   A. Proteins
   B. Carbohydrates
   C. Enzymes
   D. Lipids
   E. Porphyrins

58. Which of the following drugs typically are monitored via drug/serum blood concentrations?
   A. Theophylline
   B. Gentamicin
   C. Oxcarbazepine
   D. A and B
   E. A, B, and C

59. Which of the following has little effect on the rate of absorption of a drug?
  A. Strength
  B. pH
  C. Active transport
  D. Particle size
  E. Crystalline form

60. Enantiomers differ from one another in
  A. spatial configuration
  B. rational formula
  C. state of matter
  D. substituent groups
  E. stability

61. A compound having asymmetric carbon atoms exhibits
  A. chair-boat isomerism
  B. cis-trans isomerism
  C. optical isomerism
  D. A and B
  E. A, B, and C

62. Reduction of an aldehyde yields a (an)
  A. ketone
  B. acid
  C. peroxide
  D. primary alcohol
  E. secondary alcohol

63. Esters are formed by the reaction between
  A. acids and bases
  B. acids and alcohols
  C. acids and aldehydes
  D. acids and ketones
  E. aldehydes and bases

64. A peptide consists of
  A. two or more amino acids
  B. 20 or more amino acids
  C. an amino acid and a carbohydrate

D. an amino acid and a fat
E. an amino acid and a fatty acid

65. Tropinin I concentrations are helpful in the diagnosis of which of the following diseases?
A. Renal insufficiency
B. Acute myocardial infarctions
C. Arthritis
D. Lupus
E. Graves' disease

66. An early sign of vitamin A deficiency is
A. loss of night vision
B. a rash
C. anemia
D. pain
E. dizziness

67. Glucogenesis involves the formation of glucose from
A. noncarbohydrate sources
B. pentoses
C. aldohexoses
D. ketohexoses
E. polysaccharides

68. Primary maintenance of blood glucose between meals is due to the
A. spleen
B. liver
C. gastric mucosa
D. small intestine
E. large intestine

69. Simple lipids are esters of fatty acids with
A. glycerol
B. waxes
C. high-molecular-weight alcohols
D. low-molecular-weight alcohols
E. any alcohol

70. PSA is considered a useful marker for adenocarcinoma of the
   A. prostate
   B. breast
   C. pancreas
   D. stomach
   E. lymph nodes

71. The precursor of all steroids synthesized in the body is
   A. ATP
   B. RNA
   C. cholesterol
   D. ergosterol
   E. glycine

72. All of the following have some effect on blood glucose **EXCEPT**
   A. glucagon
   B. epinephrine
   C. thyroid hormone
   D. ACTH
   E. androgens

73. The chemical basis of heredity is
   A. acetylcholine
   B. norepinephrine
   C. RNA
   D. DNA
   E. all of the above

74. Gastrin release is increased by
   A. acetylcholine
   B. food intake
   C. elevated calcium
   D. vagal stimulation
   E. all of the above

75. Somastatin is also known as
   A. growth hormone release inhibitor
   B. secretin
   C. cholecystokinin

D. oxytocin

E. vasopressin

76. Which of the following may indicate elevated blood sodium levels?
    A. Diuretic use
    B. Dehydration
    C. Congestive heart failure
    D. A and B
    E. A, B, and C

77. Which of the following conditions may be related to increased gamma-glutamyl transferase (GGT) levels?
    A. Biliary obstruction
    B. Obstructive jaundice
    C. Cholestasis
    D. Pancreatitis
    E. All of the above

78. Absence of antidiuretic hormone in the body causes
    A. kidney failure
    B. diabetes insipidus
    C. diabetes mellitus
    D. kidney blockage
    E. hypertensive crisis

79. Bile acids are synthesized from
    A. cholesterol
    B. fatty acids
    C. acetic acid
    D. oxalic acid
    E. ATP

80. Hypercalcemia does **NOT** occur in normal individuals because
    A. calcium is rapidly excreted
    B. calcium is rapidly biotransformed
    C. calcium is insoluble
    D. excess calcium is not absorbed
    E. A and B

81. Which of the following serum levels are usually increased during hypocalcemia?
    A. Phosphate
    B. Potassium
    C. Sodium
    D. Glucose
    E. All of the above

82. Which of the following conditions are associated with increased blood ammonia levels?
    A. Reye's syndrome
    B. Liver disease
    C. Neuropathy
    D. Dermatitis
    E. Strep infections

83. Myxdema is a malfunction of which gland?
    A. Anterior pituitary
    B. Posterior pituitary
    C. Adrenal
    D. Parathyroid
    E. Thyroid

84. The primary function of the parathyroid gland is to maintain
    A. sodium balance
    B. potassium balance
    C. calcium balance
    D. bicarbonate balance
    E. electrolyte balance

85. In the male, luteinizing hormone
    A. is not present
    B. has no effect
    C. suppresses testosterone production
    D. stimulates testosterone production
    E. increases feminization

86. When oxygen binds to hemoglobin, which of the following does it displace in the normal individual?
    A. CO
    B. CO_2

C. Methyl groups
D. Iron
E. Any of the above

87. The end product of digestion of carbohydrates is (are)
   A. CO_2 and water
   B. monosaccharides
   C. glucagon
   D. glucuronic acid
   E. disaccharides

88. Which of the following is a precursor of vitamin D?
   A. Ergosterol
   B. Caprosterol
   C. Polyprenoid
   D. Cholecalciferol
   E. None of the above

89. Which of the following symptoms is most closely related to methemoglobinemia?
   A. Cyanosis
   B. Myopathy
   C. Raynaud's syndrome
   D. Chest pains
   E. Dermatitis

90. Which of the following conditions are usually measured via the D-xylose test?
   A. Malabsorption
   B. Brain tumor
   C. Glucose metabolism
   D. Renal dysfunction
   E. Thyroid function

91. The enzymes involved in ethanol metabolism are primarily
   A. phosphorylases
   B. dehydrogenases
   C. lipases
   D. ketases
   E. thiokinases

92. Amino acids that are **NOT** immediately incorporated into new protein are
  A. stored in the muscles
  B. stored in the liver
  C. recycled in the blood
  D. stored in a number of tissues
  E. rapidly degraded

93. Most nitrogenous waste is converted to urea because
  I. ammonia and uric acid are toxic
  II. urea is highly soluble
  III. urea is nontoxic

  A. I only
  B. II only
  C. I and II only
  D. II and III only
  E. I, II, and III

94. Cytochromes are useful in which reactions?
  A. Oxidation–reduction
  B. Transaminase
  C. Decarboxylation
  D. Hydrolysis
  E. Deamination

95. Acquired porphyria is usually caused by
  A. genetic defects
  B. heavy metal poisoning
  C. traumatic injury
  D. radical diets
  E. immunosuppressives

96. All of the following are true of hemolytic jaundice **EXCEPT**
  A. there is increased production of bilirubin
  B. urobilinogen concentration is increased in urine
  C. production of urobilinogen is increased
  D. bilirubin is found in the urine of the patient
  E. none of the above because all are true

97. The source of high-energy phosphate for almost every energy-requiring reaction in cells is
   A. STP
   B. DNA
   C. ATP
   D. RNA
   E. PCP

98. The end product of purine metabolism is primarily
   A. ammonia
   B. bilirubinogen
   C. bilirubin
   D. urea
   E. uric acid

99. γ-Aminobutyric acid (GABA) functions as a
   A. dehydrogenase
   B. neurotransmitter
   C. lipase
   D. amino acid precursor
   E. insulin precursor

100. A major source of folic acid is
   A. beef
   B. pork
   C. milk
   D. chicken
   E. leafy vegetables

101. A necessary precursor of visual pigment is
   A. retinal
   B. retinol
   C. ergosterol
   D. tocopherol
   E. none of the above

102. Which of the following conditions is indicative of an anion gap greater than 30 mmol/L?
A. Metabolic alkalosis
B. Metabolic acidosis
C. Urinary crystals
D. Dermatitis
E. None of the above

103. Which of the following functional groups is the most basic?
A. Amide
B. Amine
C. Aniline
D. Imide
E. Ester

104. Which of the following compounds is the most acidic?
A. Cyclohexanol
B. 4,4-Diflurocyclohexanol
C. p-Methoxyphenol
D. p-Nitrophenol
E. Phenol

105. Beta-lactams primarily undergo inactivation through
A. hydrolysis
B. isomerization
C. mutation
D. oxidation
E. reduction

106. Which of the following total serum cholesterol levels is considered desirable?
A. 300 mg/dL
B. 170 mg/dL
C. 400 mg/dL
D. 600 mg/dL
E. 250 mg/dL

107. Which of the following may be associated with hyperprolactinemia?
A. galactorrhea
B. prolactin deficiency

    C. use of antipsychotic drugs
    D. A and C
    E. A, B, and C

108. Bile acid sequesterants contain
    A. ammonium salts
    B. basic amines
    C. carboxylic acid groups
    D. mannose polymers
    E. phosphate salts

109. Conjugation of a drug substance with glucuronic acid usually occurs through which kind of linkage?
    A. Amine
    B. Ester
    C. Ether
    D. Peroxo
    E. Sulfate

110. Which of the following organ functions is assessed via testing with BUN?
    A. Cardiac
    B. Renal
    C. Ocular
    D. Liver
    E. Respiratory

111. Multidrug resistance is thought to be caused by
    A. endocytosis
    B. free-radical scavenger
    C. genetic mutation
    D. gram-negative cell wall
    E. P-glycoprotein

112. Which of the following serum concentrations is considered hyperuremia?
    A. 5 mg/dL
    B. 7 mg/dL
    C. 14 mg/dL
    D. B and C
    E. A, B, and C

113. Aldosterone causes
   A. Na⁺ retention
   B. K⁺ excretion
   C. K⁺ retention
   D. both A and B
   E. both A and C

114. Which of the following terms describes a reduced number of platelets?
   A. Thrombocytopenia
   B. Leukopenia
   C. Leukocytosis
   D. Thrombophlebitis
   E. Thrombocytosis

115. Most home pregnancy tests assay for
   A. estrogens
   B. follicle-stimulating hormone
   C. human chorionic gonadotropin
   D. luteinizing hormone–releasing hormone
   E. progestins

116. In hematologic testing, MCV is defined by the
   A. size of red blood cells
   B. amount of hemoglobin per red blood cells
   C. amount of oxygen carried by red blood cells
   D. weight of red blood cells
   E. none of the above

117. In hematologic testing, MCH is defined by the
   A. size of red blood cells
   B. percent of hemoglobin per red blood cells
   C. amount of oxygen carried by red blood cells
   D. weight of red blood cells
   E. weight of hemoglobin per average red blood cell

118. In iron deficiency anemia, which of the following indices is decreased?
   A. MCV
   B. MCH
   C. MCHC

D. A and B
E. A, B, and C

119. In hematologic testing, MCHC is defined by which of the following?
  A. size of red blood cells
  B. amount of hemoglobin per red blood cell in relation to size
  C. amount of oxygen carried by red blood cells
  D. weight of red blood cells
  E. weight of hemoglobin per average red blood cell

120. Which of the following is (are) nonhepatic causes of elevated alkaline phosphatase?
  I. Acromegaly
  II. Paget's disease
  III. Anticonvulsant drugs

  A. I only
  B. III only
  C. I and II only
  D. II and III only
  E. I, II, and III

121. Which of the following procedures are used in drug screening immunoassays?
  I. Enzyme multiplied immunoassay technique (EMIT)
  II. Radioimmunoassay (RIA)
  III. Fluorescence polarization immunoassay (FPIA)

  A. I only
  B. III only
  C. I and II only
  D. II and III only
  E. I, II, and III

122. Which of the following tests are typically included in a CBC?
  A. RBC
  B. WBC
  C. Hgb
  D. A and B
  E. A, B, and C

123. A segment of DNA that codes for a single protein is called a (an)
   A. chromosome
   B. gene
   C. intron
   D. operon
   E. ribosome

124. Creatinine clearance (CrCl) levels may be affected by
   I. age
   II. gender
   III. race

   A. I only
   B. III only
   C. I and II only
   D. II and III only
   E. I, II, and III

125. Which of the following drugs do note require monitoring via serum/plasma drug concentrations?
   A. Digoxin
   B. Warfarin
   C. Phenytoin
   D. Theophylline
   E. Cyclosporine

126. Which of the following erythromycins is least susceptible to gastric acid degradation?
   I. Estolate
   II. Base
   III. Ethylsuccinate

   A. I only
   B. III only
   C. I and II only
   D. II and III only
   E. I, II, and III

127. Toxicity is typically observed with which of the following phenytoin drug concentrations?

A. 18 (μg/mL
B. 32 (μg/mL
C. 45 (μg/mL
D. Both B and C
E. A, B, and C

128. The chemical precursor to all prostaglandins is
A. arachidonic acid
B. cholesterol
C. leukotriene
D. prostacyclin
E. thromboxane

129. For which of the following sites do parenteral aminoglycosides have good to excellent tissue penetration?
A. Prostate
B. Peritoneal fluid
C. Bone
D. Bronchial secretions
E. Pulmonary tissue

130. The levels of which kind(s) of molecules are elevated in patients with diabetes?
A. Free fatty acids
B. Ketones
C. Insulin
D. Both A and B
E. A, B, and C

131. Clinical uses for monitoring creatinine clearance (CrCl) and serum creatinine (SCr) include
I. assessing kidney function in acute renal failure patients
II. monitoring patients on nephrotoxic drugs
III. determining dosage adjustments for renally eliminated drugs

A. I only
B. III only
C. I and II only
D. II and III only
E. I, II, and III

132. False-positive urine drug screens may be attributed to
   I. chemical structure similarity between substances tested for and medication taken by patient
   II. foodstuffs taken 24 hours prior to test
   III. heating urine before analysis

   A. I only
   B. III only
   C. I and II only
   D. II and III only
   E. I, II, and III

133. Carcinoembryonic antigen (CEA) is a marker for which of the following carcinomas?
   I. Colorectal
   II. Breast
   III. Gastrointestinal

   A. I only
   B. III only
   C. I and II only
   D. II and III only
   E. I, II, and III

134. The measurement of C-peptide exhibits a number of advantages compared to peripheral insulin measurement, including which of the following?
   I. C-peptide levels are better indicators of β-cell function
   II. C-peptide assays do not react with insulin antibodies
   III. C-peptide measurement is heat resistant

   A. I only
   B. III only
   C. I and II only
   D. II and III only
   E. I, II, and III

135. Lactic acid is predominantly derived from which of the following area(s)?
  I. Skeletal muscle
  II. Brain
  III. Erythrocytes

  A. I only
  B. III only
  C. I and II only
  D. II and III only
  E. I, II, and III

136. Which of the following conditions may be associated with increased levels of serum eosinophils?
  I. Allergic reaction to latex
  II. Drug hypersensitivity reaction
  III. Parasitic infestation

  A. I only
  B. III only
  C. I and II only
  D. II and III only
  E. I, II, and III

137. MRI uses the same principle as
  A. HPLC
  B. IR
  C. NMR
  D. UV
  E. UV-vis

138. Which of the following have been associated with hypercalcemia?
  I. Malignant tumors
  II. Primary hyperparathyroidisms
  III. Thiazide diuretics

  A. I only
  B. III only
  C. I and II only
  D. II and III only
  E. I, II, and III

139. The prothrombin time test measures deficiencies in which of the following factors?
  I. Prothrombin (factor II)
  II. Factor IX
  III. Factor XII

  A. I only
  B. III only
  C. I and II only
  D. II and III only
  E. I, II, and III

140. The current guidelines of the American College of Chest Physicians' and National Heart, Lung and Blood Institute recommend that an INR for all indications (excluding mechanical prosthetic heart valves) be in which of the following ranges?
  A. 1.0–1.5
  B. 1.5–2.5
  C. 2.0–3.0
  D. 2.5–3.5
  E. 3.0–4.0

Chemistry and Biochemistry

Answers and Discussion

1. **(C)** Amiloride, spironolactone, and triamterene are all potassium-sparing diuretics.

2. **(B)** Sodium polysterene sulfonate removes potassium by exchanging sodium ions for potassium ions in the intestines before the resin is passed from the body. Exchange capacity is 1 mEq/g in vivo and 3.1 mEq/g in vitro.

3. **(A)** Aspirin hydrolyzes to salicylic acid and acetic acid.

4. **(E)** Grignard reagents are R—Mg—X compounds that are used as intermediates in synthesis.

5. **(C)** NMR is based on the fact that different molecular arrangements have different magnetic spin characteristics.

6. **(B)** Na_2SO_4 is the formula; substances react in a 2:1 ratio.

7. **(A)** Calcium carbonate contains the highest percentage of elemental calcium (40%) as compared to the salts of citrate (21%), glubionate (6.5%), gluconate (9.3%), and lactate (13%).

8. **(C)** Hypokalemia is a potential side effect of the other drugs mentioned, except for ACE inhibitors, which have

been associated with hyperkalemia (incidence up to 11% with some drugs in this class).

9. **(E)** Adsorption can be either reversible or irreversible, and is not a chemical reaction.

10. **(A)** This group is widely used for general anesthesia because of its lack of flammability.

11. **(D)** Hydrolyzation produces amino acids.

12. **(D)** All of the statements are true except that this agent must be prepared in a radiopharmaceutical area.

13. **(C)** This is obtained by dividing molecule weight by hydrogen equivalent.

14. **(B)** Aluminum hydroxide and its salts coat the stomach.

15. **(D)** Both alcohol groups are oxidized completely and form HOOC—COOH, which is oxalic acid.

16. **(A)** The ANA test lacks specificity but is often seen in the diagnosis of rheumatic diseases, particularly systemic lupus erythematosus.

17. **(C)** Primary alcohols are oxidized to aldehydes or acids. Tertiary alcohols are not oxidized and there are no quarternary alcohols.

18. **(E)** Functional groups determine water and lipid solubility and reactivity, as well as chemical and/or in vivo stability.

19. **(B)** The OH group is an alcohol, the COOH group is an acid, and the R—O—R is an ether.

20. **(A)** Cellulose is a polysaccharide found in plant cell walls and cannot be digested by humans.

21. **(C)** BAL chelates mercury, gold, antimony, and arsenic, and renders them insoluble and less toxic or nontoxic.

22. **(A)**   Only iodides are used for expectorant action in cough syrups.

23. **(B)**   Strontium has an affinity for bone and is used to study bone lesions or abnormal structures in bone.

24. **(A)**   Penicillamine chelates lead, copper, and other heavy metals to form stable, soluble complexes that are excreted in the urine.

25. **(A)**   Only repeated distillation ensures sterility and lack of pyrogen contaminants.

26. **(C)**   Sorbic acid is fungistatic and is used to inhibit yeasts or molds.

27. **(B)**   Silver salt solutions form insoluble AgCl. The others are soluble and compatible.

28. **(A)**   All are members of group O (inert gases) except nitrogen, which is a member of group V-A of the periodic table.

29. **(E)**   Zirconium salts are useful in treating poison ivy, oak, or sumac.

30. **(D)**   Vitamin K is not an antioxidant.

31. **(D)**   Mannitol crystallizes very easily. Thus, to prevent these crystals from being administered to the patient, a filter should be used during administration.

32. **(A)**   Ascorbic acid is unstable to any increase in temperature, particularly in the presence of metals.

33. **(D)**   Of the 10 essential amino acids, glutamine is not included.

34. **(C)**   Tyramine is normally destroyed by MAO.

35. **(A)**   The ferrous ion in the nitroprusside molecule reacts rapidly with sulfhydryl compounds in red blood cells, which results in the release of cyanide.

36. (D) The physiologic heat of combustion of fats is more than twice that of proteins or carbohydrates.

37. (B) Pepsinogen is a precursor; the other choices are not found in gastric juice.

38. (A) A fasting blood glucose concentration is the best indicator of glucose homeostasis. Normal range is 70–110 mg/dL. Values >140 mg/dL found on at least two separate occasions indicate glucose intolerance.

39. (D) Concomitant phenobarbital and warfarin therapy has been reported to result in decreased anticoagulant effect, primarily due to induction of hepatic metabolism of warfarin.

40. (B) Starch is a disaccharide formed only in the mammary glands.

41. (C) Glycogen is converted to D-glucose.

42. (C) Vitamin A aldehydes are components of visual purple.

43. (A) Lipids and albuminoids are not usually present.

44. (C) Vitamin K mediates prothrombin formation and aids clotting.

45. (E) ATP provides the energy for contraction.

46. (E) Both hormones affect the growth and development of the gonads.

47. (E) Insulin is a hormone and a protein that is produced by the pancreas (specifically the islets of Langerhans), and is distributed primarily in extracellular fluids.

48. (E) The range is from 90–140 days. The life span is determined by tagging with radioactive tracers.

49. (D) Thyroglobulin is found in the thyroid glands. It has many reactive tyrosyl residues.

50. **(B)** B complex and C are mainly water soluble.

51. **(C)** Vitamin B_{12} is a generic term for several cobalt-containing compounds, designated cobalamins. The R group attached to the central cobalt atom determines the type of vitamin B_{12} congener (cyano group in cyanocobalamin, hydroxy group in hydroxocobalamin, methyl group in methylcobalamin, and deoxyadenosyl group in deoxyadenosylcobalamin).

52. **(D)** Zinc deficiency results in retardation of growth.

53. **(C)** Cyanide inactivates this respiratory enzyme.

54. **(E)** Levels of more than 7.5 mg% usually produce severe symptoms.

55. **(C)** Stimulation of these enzymes may decrease blood levels and efficacy of other drugs given concurrently.

56. **(E)** Ribose or desoxyribose is the carbohydrate portion.

57. **(D)** They all are 20-carbon–atom fatty acids.

58. **(D)** Both gentamicin and theophylline are typically monitored via serum concentrations. Therapeutic ranges for theophylline range from 10–20 µg/mL and peak ranges for gentamicin range from 6–10 µg/mL depending on the site and severity of infection. Using drug concentrations to monitor oxcarbazepine has not been established.

59. **(A)** The strength might have some effect if solubility is exceeded; the other choices have many more side effects.

60. **(A)** Enantiomers differ only in the way the atoms are oriented in space.

61. **(C)** Compounds with asymmetric carbon atoms exhibit only optical isomerism. Chair-boat or cis-trans isomerism is based on double-bond linkages.

62. **(D)** Because aldehydes have a single alkyl group attached, they are reduced to primary alcohols.

63. (B) The general reaction is between acids and alcohols: $RCOOH + ROH \rightarrow RCOOR + H_2O$.

64. (A) A peptide consists of two or more amino acids linked by peptide bonds. If there is a residue of 10 or more amino acids, it is a polypeptide.

65. (B) Tropinin I is useful in the diagnosis of acute myocardial infarctions (MI) with similar sensitivity to CK-MB levels from 4–8 hours post MI.

66. (A) Vitamin A is necessary for vision; night vision is most sensitive to a deficiency. Other symptoms are not seen.

67. (A) The principal substrates are amino acids, lactate, and glycerol. All of the others are carbohydrates.

68. (B) The liver is the chief source of glycogen to maintain blood glucose. The muscle uses its glycogen to support muscle activity.

69. (D) Simple lipids are esters made from lower-molecular-weight alcohols of various types.

70. (A) Prostate specific antigen (PSA) is increased in men with significant prostate cancer. The use of this test increases rate of detection. PSA is a protease produced exclusively by prostate epithelial cells. It may be increased during instrumentation or local surgery.

71. (C) The original building block is cholesterol. Ergosterol comes from plant sources.

72. (E) All except androgens play a role in blood glucose levels.

73. (D) DNA contains all the genetic information affecting heredity.

74. (E) Gastrin release is increased by all of the factors or substances listed.

75. **(A)**   Somostatin is a regulator of growth hormone, insulin, and glycogen secretion.

76. **(D)**   Diuretic use and dehydration are often common causes of hypernatremia. CHF is often associated with hyponatremia.

77. **(E)**   GGT is a biliary excretory enzyme useful in the diagnosis of certain liver diseases, including cholestatic and obstructive jaundice.

78. **(B)**   Diabetes insipidus results in and is characterized by massive urine flow.

79. **(A)**   Bile acids are synthesized from cholesterol in a multistep process.

80. **(D)**   Excess calcium simply is not absorbed when adequate levels are present in normal persons.

81. **(A)**   Serum phosphate levels tend to be increased when serum calcium levels are decreased.

82. **(B)**   The diagnostic utility of ammonia levels are limited but they may be indicative of cirrhosis and poor liver function.

83. **(E)**   Myxedema, also known as hypothyroidism, is caused by an insufficiency of thyroid hormones.

84. **(C)**   Parathyroid hormone regulates the concentration of ionized calcium within a narrow range.

85. **(D)**   Luteinizing hormone stimulates testosterone production, which in turn aids spermatogenesis.

86. **(B)**   Oxygen displaces CO_2, which is exhaled. Iron is a part of heme and CO; the other entities are not present normally.

87. **(B)**   The hydrolytic processes produce monosaccharides (principally glucose).

88. (A) Irradiation of UV light causes conversion. Calciferol is vitamin D.

89. (A) Methemoglobinemia is caused by the oxidation of the reduced ferrous (Fe^{2+}) iron of hemoglobin to the ferric (Fe^{3+}) form, making it incapable of binding oxygen for transport. Thus, cyanosis is a typical symptom.

90. (A) The use of the D-xylose test is primarily related to malabsorption syndromes such as tropical sprue, and celiac disease. It is a test to assess the functional integrity of the jejunum.

91. (B) These are oxidizing enzymes known as alcohol dehydrogenase and aldehyde dehydrogenase.

92. (E) Excessive amino acids are not stored, and they are rapidly degraded.

93. (E) Humans and other mammals have evolved in their capacity to get rid of toxic ammonia and insoluble uric acid as soluble, nontoxic urea.

94. (A) Cytochromes act as transfer agents in oxidation–reduction reactions.

95. (B) Acquired porphyria is usually due to lead or heavy metal poisoning or the drugs griseofulvin or apronalide.

96. (D) In spite of increased production of bilirubin, it is not usually found in the urine in hemolytic jaundice.

97. (C) Adenosine triphosphate (ATP) is extremely important to cells as a high-energy phosphate source.

98. (E) The end product is primarily uric acid or its salts. The salts are much more soluble.

99. (B) GABA is a neurotransmitter formed from glutamate in brain tissue.

100. (E) Animal cells cannot synthesize PABA, which constitutes a portion of folic acid.

101. (A) Retinol is a hormone. All the others except retinal are unrelated to vitamin A, which generates rhodopsin (pigment).

102. (B) Anion gap represents the approximate sum of measured anions minus unmeasured cations (anion gap = Na^+ − [Cl^- +HCO_3^-]). When increased, it may indicate lactic acidosis or ketoacidosis.

103. (B) Amines are more basic than any of the sp-2 hybridized forms or those capable of resonance into a carbonyl.

104. (D) The para-nitro group can withdraw electrons via resonance.

105. (C) β-Lactamases are enzymes that open the β-lactam ring.

106. (B) Target total cholesterol levels are <200 mg/dL.

107. (D) Hyperprolactinemia is typically associated with clinical symptoms of galactorrhea and may often be caused by use of several types of antipsychotic agents.

108. (A) Bile acid sequestrants contain either quaternary ammonium salts or HCl salts of a tertiary amine.

109. (B) Alcohols are conjugated by condensation with the C-6 carboxylic acid group of glucuronic acid.

110. (B) BUN testing is used to assess renal function, particularly in combination with serum creatinine values.

111. (E) The protein causes cellular efflux of a variety of drugs.

112. (C) Uric acid levels >12.0 mg/dL are considered hyperuricemia and may be related to conditions of gout.

113. (C) Aldosterone both promotes sodium reabsorption and potassium excretion by action at the distal tubule of the kidney.

114. (A) A decreased number of platelets is usually referred to as thrombocytopenia.

115. (C) Most home pregnancy tests measure levels of human chorionic gonadotropin. This agent is produced by a fertilized ovum and has essentially the same effects as LHRH.

116. (A) Mean corpuscular volume (MCV) refers to the size (volume) of red blood cells.

117. (E) Mean cell hemoglobin (MCH) refers to the weight of hemoglobin in the average red blood cell.

118. (E) All of the indices are decreased in iron deficiency anemia.

119. (B) MCHC (mean corpuscular hemoglobin concentration) refers to the amount of hemoglobin in the average red blood cell in relation to its size.

120. (E) Alkaline phosphatase (ALP) is a group of enzymes in many body tissues, including the liver, bone, small intestine, and kidneys, as well as plasma and leukocytes. Bone disorders such as Paget's disease, anticonvulsants (i.e., phenytoin, phenobarbital), and acromegaly can all cause general increases in ALP.

121. (E) All of these immunoassays are common screening tests. EMIT is used by all National Institute on Drug Abuse (NIDA) certified laboratories. RIA is used for urine testing for nonforensic purposes. FPIA is the most common form of immunoassay.

122. (E) A CBC traditionally includes RBC count, WBC count, Hgb, HCT, RBC indices, reticulocyte count, RBC distribution width, and platelet count.

123. (B)   A gene is defined as a section of DNA corresponding to a single protein.

124. (C)   Age and gender are two important factors affecting CrCl. CrCl declines with age even with a "normal" serum creatinine value. In females, the CrCl is usually 93% of that measured in males.

125. (D)   All of the named drugs require serum/plasma or blood drug monitoring except warfarin which is monitored via clotting testing.

126. (A)   Estolate is the most acid-stable erythromycin product.

127. (D)   Phenytoin levels above 20 µg/mL may be associated with symptoms of toxicity.

128. (A)   Leukotriene, prostacyclin, and thromboxane are derived from arachidonic acid through oxidation.

129. (E)   Tissue penetration is poor for all the sites mentioned with the exception of pulmonary tissue.

130. (D)   Both fatty acids and ketone bodies are characteristics of diabetes mellitus.

131. (E)   All of these listed are common clinical uses. The relationship between SCr and CrCl is inverse and geometric as opposed to linear.

132. (C)   Most urine drug screens test for general chemical structure and thus may be prone to false-positive results if other substances are in urine that share a similar chemical structure. Some foodstuffs, such as poppy seeds, have been documented to produce false-positive opiate screening test results.

133. (E)   CEA is a glycoprotein. In the healthy population, the upper limit of CEA is about 3 ng/L for nonsmokers and about 5 ng/L for smokers. This is a nonspecific marker for certain types of carcinoma, including colorectal, breast, gastrointestinal, pancreatic, ovarian, and uterine. In breast cancer, an elevated CEA usually indicates metastatic disease.

134. (C) Within the pancreatic b-cells, proinsulin is cleaved to produce insulin and C-peptide. C-peptide levels are better indicators of b-cell function because they undergo minimal liver metabolism and do not react with anti-insulin antibodies.

135. (E) Lactic acid is an intermediary in carbohydrate metabolism and is derived from all three: skeletal muscle, brain, and erythrocytes.

136. (E) Eosinophilia may indicate an allergic reaction, a drug sensitivity reaction, or a parasitic infestation.

137. (C) Both techniques use involve magnetic resonance techniques.

138. (E) Osteolytic metastases can increase serum calcium via bone invasion and subsequent degradation of bone matrix and mineral content. Primary hyperparathyroidism may increase serum calcium via inappropriate secretion of PTH from the parathyroid gland. Approximately 2% of patients treated with thiazide diuretics may develop hypercalcemia.

139. (C) PT measures deficiencies in factors II and IX.

140. (C) Current ACCP and NHLBI guidelines recommend an INR of 2.0–3.0 for all indications except mechanical prosthetic heart valves, for which an INR of 2.5–3.5 is recommended.

5

Physiology and Pathology

DIRECTIONS (Questions 1–95): Each of the questions or incomplete statements below is followed by five suggested answers or completions. Select the **one answer** that is best in each case.

1. A patient in a diabetic coma
   A. may have the odor of acetone on his breath
   B. may be perspiring profusely
   C. usually recovers without treatment
   D. may twitch excessively
   E. none of the above

2. One of the most potent stimulants of the respiratory center is
   A. increased P_{O_2} in the blood
   B. decreased P_{O_2} in the blood
   C. increased P_{CO_2} in the blood
   D. decreased P_{CO_2} in the blood
   E. none of the above

3. The P wave on the electrocardiogram is associated with
   A. atrial repolarization
   B. atrial contraction
   C. atrial depolarization
   D. ventricular repolarization
   E. none of the above

4. The A wave of the venous pulse is caused by
   A. atrial contraction that impedes blood flow in the large veins
   B. incoming blood that stagnates during ventricular systole
   C. the thrust of the blood into the aorta that is transmitted to the large veins
   D. an abnormally constricted vena cava
   E. none of the above

5. The disintegration of the platelets gives rise to a factor required for normal blood coagulation. This factor is
   A. thromboplastin
   B. thrombin
   C. prothrombin
   D. fibrinogen
   E. none of the above

6. Drugs that stimulate the parasympathetic branch of the autonomic nervous system are called
   A. anticholinergics
   B. adrenergic agents
   C. cholinergic agents
   D. cholinolytic agents
   E. sympathomimetics

7. The respiratory center is located in the
   A. cerebrum
   B. cerebellum
   C. hypothalamus
   D. medulla
   E. pons

8. Cerebral transient ischemic attacks frequently present which of the following symptoms?
   A. "Pins and needles" numbness in limb
   B. Weakness of lower face, hand, or limb
   C. Dysphasia
   D. Blurred vision
   E. All of the above

9. Cerebellar corticol degeneration is often associated with
   A. pregnancy
   B. alcohol abuse
   C. obesity
   D. loud music
   E. all of the above

10. What is the primary function of the colon?
    A. Digestion
    B. Mastication
    C. Collection of urine
    D. Reabsorption of water and electrolytes
    E. Separation of urine from feces

11. The primary function of gastrointestinal villi is to
    A. facilitate the passage of chyme through the GI tract
    B. increase the surface area of the GI tract
    C. debride food particles into smaller sizes
    D. break down amino acids into smaller molecules
    E. A and C

12. A lipoma is
    A. produced by sweat glands
    B. a cancerous lump of the lymph glands
    C. a fatty tumor
    D. only found in the bloodstream
    E. A and B

13. Which of the following is (are) secreted by the pancreas?
    A. Insulin
    B. FSH
    C. Glucagon
    D. ACTH
    E. A and C

14. Amenorrhea may be defined as
    A. painful menstruation
    B. premenstrual syndrome
    C. impotence
    D. absence of menstruation
    E. cystic acne

15. What type of anemia is caused by iron deficiency?
   A. Macrocytic, hypochromic
   B. Microcytic, normochromic
   C. Macrocytic
   D. Normochromic, normocytic
   E. Microcytic, hypochromic

16. In young adults, normal blood pressure is
   A. 100/60
   B. 80/80
   C. 140/90
   D. 120/120
   E. 120/80

17. Systemic diastolic pressure depends largely on
   A. cardiac output
   B. elasticity
   C. peripheral resistance
   D. A and B
   E. B and C

18. The glomerulus is
   A. a network of capillaries
   B. a lymph node
   C. a large artery entering the kidney
   D. a dilator substance produced by the kidney
   E. none of the above

19. Henle's loop is found in the
   A. liver
   B. stomach
   C. intestine
   D. kidney
   E. inner ear

20. A lack of speech coordination is
   A. dysphasia
   B. paresthesia
   C. dyspnea
   D. diplopia
   E. dyspraxia

21. The fundamental unit of organized neural activity is the
    A. ganglion
    B. reflex arc
    C. synapse
    D. afferent neuron
    E. efferent neuron

22. Antidiuretic hormone is secreted from
    A. the kidney cortex
    B. the kidney medulla
    C. the anterior pituitary
    D. the posterior pituitary
    E. none of the above

23. The sympathetic ganglia are located
    A. near the heart
    B. near the spinal cord
    C. near the adrenal glands
    D. near the tissues they innervate
    E. in the extremities

24. The chemical mediator released at the end of the parasympathetic nerve fiber is
    A. acetylcholine esterase
    B. acetylcholine
    C. epinephrine
    D. norepinephrine
    E. amino oxidase

25. An endocrine gland that plays an important role in calcium metabolism is the
    A. pancreas
    B. hypophysis
    C. thyroid
    D. parathyroid
    E. gonads

26. Heat cramps are due primarily to loss of
    A. water
    B. body temperature
    C. lithium
    D. potassium
    E. sodium

27. The most important functional process that the neutrophils and monocytes carry out is
    A. phagocytosis
    B. IDK
    C. tachyphylaxis
    D. urea absorption
    E. none of the above

28. The uppermost portion of the intestine is the
    A. cecum
    B. jejunum
    C. ileum
    D. duodenum
    E. colon

29. The pigment that gives the urine its color is
    A. urochrome
    B. bilirubin
    C. biliverdin
    D. urobilin
    E. none of the above

30. Equalization of air pressure between the tympanic cavity and the outside atmosphere is done by the
    A. stapes
    B. cochlea
    C. eustachian tube
    D. anvil
    E. semicircular canal

31. The neurotransmitter released at the end of the sympathetic nerve fiber is
    A. epinephrine
    B. norepinephrine

    C. acetylcholine
    D. acetylcholine esterase
    E. amine oxidase

32. Drugs that cause dilation of the eye pupil are
    A. miotics
    B. mydriatics
    C. cycloplegics
    D. antispasmodics
    E. anorectics

33. The most common blood type is
    A. A
    B. B
    C. O
    D. AB
    E. X

34. Which of the following products stimulates the production of red blood cells?
    A. Erythropoietin
    B. Filgrastim
    C. Sargramostim
    D. Oprelvekin
    E. None of the above

35. The bundles of His are found in the
    A. lung
    B. intestines
    C. liver
    D. heart
    E. kidneys

36. The pacemaker of the heart is the
    A. coronary artery
    B. right ventricle
    C. SA node
    D. AV node
    E. left ventricle

37. Rales are
   A. lesions
   B. visual disturbances
   C. flashing pains
   D. abnormal chest sounds
   E. none of the above

38. Hodgkin's disease is usually centered in the
   A. central nervous system
   B. GI system
   C. musculoskeletal system
   D. lymphatic system
   E. blood

39. The principal action of the lymph glands is
   A. to destroy microorganisms
   B. to be a warning system
   C. to reduce fever
   D. to filter out solids
   E. none of the above

40. Diverticulosis is usually associated with the
   A. stomach
   B. small intestine
   C. liver
   D. skin
   E. colon

41. The sensory ganglion of the brain stem is the
   A. cerebral cortex
   B. hypothalamus
   C. thalamus
   D. medulla
   E. basal ganglia

42. Which of the following are a result of proton pump inhibition?
   A. Decreased gastric acid secretion
   B. Decreased gastric histamine release
   C. Increased gastric acid secretion
   D. Anticholinergic action
   E. None of the above

43. When light rays come to a focus behind the retina, the eye is said to be
   A. hypermetropic
   B. presbyopic
   C. astigmatic
   D. myopic
   E. emmetropic

44. Progressive fibrosis and scarring of the liver are known as
   A. diverticulitis
   B. diverticulosis
   C. hepatitis
   D. cirrhosis
   E. ulcerative colitis

45. Major constituents of bile are
   A. nonelectrolytes
   B. organic acids
   C. organic bases
   D. micelles
   E. inorganic bases

46. Histoplasmosis is caused by an internal invasion of the body by
   A. viruses
   B. fungi
   C. helminths
   D. bacteria
   E. rickettsia

47. The ion in highest concentration in the cells is
   A. Na
   B. Mg
   C. K
   D. Ca
   E. Fe

48. The ion in highest concentration outside the cells is
  A. Na
  B. Mg
  C. K
  D. Ca
  E. Fe

49. Heavy metals exert their toxic effects in the body by
  A. blocking enzymes
  B. sclerosing tissues
  C. precipitating proteins
  D. depressing oxygen exchange
  E. none of the above

50. A term denoting dryness of the mouth is
  A. zerophthalmia
  B. stomatitis
  C. xerostomia
  D. xerotocia
  E. xeromenia

51. Polycythemia is characterized by
  A. anemia
  B. high white blood cell count
  C. high red blood cell count
  D. low red blood cell count
  E. eosinophilia

52. Bilirubin is produced by
  A. biosynthesis
  B. the kidneys
  C. hemoglobin decomposition
  D. decomposition of bile salts
  E. the spleen

53. Which of the following transport(s) urine to the bladder?
  A. Urethra
  B. Ureters
  C. Glomeruli
  D. Loop of Henle
  E. None of the above

54. The main function of the gallbladder is to
   A. secrete bile
   B. concentrate bile
   C. eliminate bile
   D. biosynthesize bile
   E. do none of the above

55. Crohn's disease is a disease of the
   A. brain
   B. spinal cord
   C. stomach
   D. colon
   E. kidney

56. The most prevalent type of white blood cells are the
   A. lymphocytes
   B. eosinophils
   C. basophils
   D. neutrophils
   E. monocytes

57. Secretion of adrenal cortical hormones is controlled primarily by
   A. somatotropic hormone
   B. epinephrine
   C. glucagon
   D. ACTH
   E. ICSH

58. Most patients suffer from acute renal failure as a result of
   A. dehydration
   B. nitrosis
   C. cirrhosis
   D. bacterial infection
   E. hyperkalemia

59. Tourette's syndrome is a disorder that typically presents with which of the following symptoms?
   A. Verbal and motor tics
   B. Dysphagia
   C. Myopathy
   D. Dermatitis
   E. None of the above

60. An inflammation of the kidney substance and pelvis is
   A. pyelonephritis
   B. hepatitis
   C. pyemesis
   D. pyometritis
   E. perichondritis

61. A wasting due to lack of nutrition to a body part is
   A. atrophy
   B. hypertrophy
   C. aplasia
   D. hyperplasia
   E. gerontopia

62. The breast bone is called the
   A. sternum
   B. thorax
   C. ribs
   D. ulna
   E. femur

63. Dyspnea means
   A. painful muscle spasm
   B. pain in the heart
   C. pain in extremities
   D. painful breathing
   E. none of the above

64. Sickle cell anemia is characterized by
   A. lack of iron
   B. lack of B_{12}
   C. abnormally shaped red blood cells
   D. lack of folic acid
   E. megaloblastic red blood cells

65. Graves' disease may be characterized by
   A. hepatic cirrhosis
   B. hypothyroidism
   C. cortisol insufficiency
   D. hyperthyroidism
   E. glomerulonephritis

66. REM is an essential component of the sleep cycle. This period, characterized by rapid eye movement, is also referred to as
   A. deep sleep
   B. restful sleep
   C. dream sleep
   D. insomniac sleep
   E. cell repair sleep

67. Narcolepsy is a disease is manifested by which of the following symptoms?
   A. Insomnia
   B. Sudden sleep attacks
   C. Hiccups
   D. Bruising
   E. Pulmonary infections

68. Which of the following defines parasitosis?
   A. Delusions of parasite infestations
   B. Parasite infestation with tape worms
   C. Infestation with ticks or fleas
   D. Infestation with fungal organism
   E. None of the above

69. Hepatitis may be detected by
   A. the presence of jaundice
   B. elevated AST
   C. elevated ALT
   D. elevated bilirubin
   E. all of the above

70. Thyrotoxicosis is characterized by
   A. excessive thyroid hormone
   B. insufficient thyroid hormone
   C. an infection of the hypothalamus
   D. an atrophied thyroid gland
   E. B and D

71. Raynaud's syndrome is caused by which of the following actions?
   A. Digital vasodilatation
   B. Digital vasoconstriction
   C. Hyperglycemia
   D. Hypoglycemia
   E. None of the above

72. Lipodystrophy is often seen in
   A. hepatitis
   B. hyperthyroidism
   C. insulin-dependent diabetes
   D. young children
   E. women of childbearing age

73. The parathyroid is responsible for
   A. calcium metabolism
   B. secretion of thyroid hormones
   C. maintaining the parasympathetic nervous system
   D. cardiac output
   E. pulmonary function

74. Vitamin B_{12} is absorbed by complexation with intrinsic factor. Intrinsic factor may be described as
   A. enzyme
   B. carbohydrate
   C. lipid
   D. glycoprotein
   E. penetration enhancer

75. The manifestations of myasthenia gravis are due to
   A. hypertonicity of smooth muscle
   B. weakness of striated muscle
   C. hypertonicity of striated muscle

   D. weakness of smooth muscle
   E. sclerosis of striated muscle

76. In open angle glaucoma, the increase in intraocular pressure is caused by
   A. angle closure
   B. physical blockage of the trabecular network
   C. excessive production of aqueous humor
   D. large eyeballs
   E. all of the above

77. In psoriatic conditions, all turnover time is
   A. reduced to 4–5 days
   B. increased to 30–60 days
   C. unchanged
   D. increased 4-fold
   E. reduced one-third

78. Toxic shock syndrome is characterized by sudden onset of
   A. high fever
   B. rash on palms and soles
   C. dizziness
   D. nausea, vomiting, and diarrhea
   E. all of the above

79. Conjunctivitis may be caused by
   A. foreign bodies
   B. allergies
   C. chemical burns
   D. infection
   E. all of the above

80. Vaginal candidiasis is common in
   I. pregnant women
   II. women taking broad spectrum antibiotics
   III. diabetic women

   A. I only
   B. III only
   C. I and II only
   D. II and III only
   E. I, II, and III

81. Possible causes of secondary hypertension include
    I. renal disease
    II. oral decongestants
    III. fenfluramine

    A. I only
    B. III only
    C. I and II only
    D. II and III only
    E. I, II, and III

82. Cardiac output is the product of ventricular stroke volume and
    A. diastolic pressure
    B. ventricular wall tension
    C. left ventricular ejection fraction
    D. heart rate
    E. inotropic rate

83. If coronary blood flow is significantly obstructed by atherosclerotic plaques, a patient is most likely to develop symptoms of
    A. hypertension
    B. headaches
    C. angina
    D. pulmonary edema
    E. peripheral edema

84. Vitamin K is essential in the formation of clotting factor(s)
    I. factor II
    II. factor IX
    III. factor X

    A. I only
    B. III only
    C. I and II only
    D. II and III only
    E. I, II, and III

85. Hyperresponsiveness of the trachea and bronchi to stimuli with bronchiolar constriction and symptoms of wheezing and dyspnea describes
   A. chronic bronchitis
   B. asthma
   C. pneumonia
   D. chronic obstructive pulmonary disease
   E. upper respiratory tract infection

86. Which of the following drugs is (are) known to cause pulmonary fibrosis?
   I. Bleomycin
   II. Aspirin
   III. Amiodarone

   A. I only
   B. III only
   C. I and II only
   D. II and III only
   E. I, II, and III

87. Which of the following factors increases the risk of pneumonia?
   I. Chronic allergic rhinitis
   II. Use of broad spectrum antibiotics in a patient in a nursing home
   III. Stroke or head injuries

   A. I only
   B. III only
   C. I and II only
   D. II and III only
   E. I, II, and III

88. *Helicobacter pylori* infection is associated with
   A. peptic ulcer disease
   B. pseudomembranous colitis
   C. otitis media
   D. Crohn's disease
   E. pyelonephritis

89. A normal creatinine clearance for an adult male is
   A. 24 mL/min
   B. 72 mL/min
   C. 120 mL/min
   D. 250 mL/min
   E. 662 mL/min

90. Tinea versicolor is
   A. athlete's foot
   B. a photoallergic skin reaction
   C. an inflammation of the eardrum
   D. a fungal infection of the stratum corneum
   E. a viral infection of the nail bed

91. The layer of skin that has the greatest effect on percutaneous absorption of drugs is
   A. stratum spinosum
   B. subcutaneous layer
   C. stratum germinatum
   D. dermis
   E. stratum corneum

92. In psoriasis, epidermal cells
   I. proliferate at a rate 7–10 times faster than normal cells
   II. are resistant to phototherapy
   III. are very thin and friable

   A. I only
   B. III only
   C. I and II only
   D. II and III only
   E. I, II, and III

93. The outer layer of the eye is composed of the
   I. sclera
   II. conjunctiva
   III. cornea

   A. I only
   B. III only
   C. I and II only

D. II and III only
E. I, II, and III

94. Patients with non–insulin-dependent diabetes mellitus (NIDDM) usually have
I. tissue resistance to insulin
II. a reduced number of insulin receptors
III. circulating islet cell antibodies

A. I only
B. III only
C. I and II only
D. II and III only
E. I, II, and III

95. The **MOST** likely cause(s) of ventricular arrhythmias is (are)
I. potassium depletion
II. hyperkalemia
III. magnesium depletion

A. I only
B. III only
C. I and II only
D. II and III only
E. I, II, and III

Physiology and Pathology

Answers and Discussion

1. **(A)** The odor of acetone is due to ketoacidosis.

2. **(C)** Increased P_{CO_2} in the blood triggers the respiratory center to increase respiration to produce exchange.

3. **(C)** The P wave is the record of atrial depolarization.

4. **(A)** The A wave is a record of the resistance encountered.

5. **(A)** It also releases other thromboplastic factors.

6. **(C)** Cholinergic agents are mediated by acetylcholine.

7. **(D)** All of the vital centers are located in the medulla.

8. **(E)** All of these symptoms may be present and are indicative of the area of the brain that is damaged.

9. **(B)** Cerebral corticol degenerations is often referred to as alcoholic cerebellar degeneration that has occurred as a chronic nutritional depletion. A history of chronic alcoholism is commonly associated with poor eating habits, which produce malnutrition.

10. **(D)** The body strives to conserve useful electrolytes and water; this reabsorption occurs in the colon. As a result of this function, fecal material is also concentrated.

11. **(B)** Increasing the surface area with tiny projections like the villi provides increased sites for absorption of nutrients.

12. **(C)** A lipoma is generally a benign tumor consisting of a collection of fatty cells.

13. **(E)** Glucagon and insulin are both secreted by the pancreas. Beta cells release insulin and alpha cells release glucagon.

14. **(D)** An absence of menstruation may be attributed to unresponsiveness of the endometrium due to inadequate production of gonadotrophins, adrenal disease, ovarian dysfunction, or pregnancy.

15. **(E)** Iron is necessary for hemoglobin synthesis. Decreased amounts of hemoglobin cause erythrocytes to be small and lightly colored.

16. **(E)** Blood pressure varies from one individual to another and is only a rough estimate.

17. **(E)** Elasticity is closely tied to peripheral resistance.

18. **(A)** The glomerulus contains up to 50 parallel capillaries encased in Bowman's capsule, in which fluid collects.

19. **(D)** It is the area between the proximal and distal tubules.

20. **(A)** Dysphasia is usually correctable by speech therapy.

21. **(B)** The key word is *organized.*

22. **(D)** The hypothalamus also is involved.

23. **(B)** They are autonomic ganglia.

24. (B) Epinephrine and norepinephrine are released in the sympathetic system, and the two enzymes are not mediators.

25. (D) This is the chief function of the parathyroid gland.

26. (E) Heat cramps are caused by loss of sodium through sweating.

27. (A) Neutrophils and monocytes are types of white blood cells.

28. (D) The stomach empties directly into the duodenum. The ileum and jejunum are lower.

29. (A) The others may change the basic color, however.

30. (C) Failure to equalize may cause pain and require myringotomy.

31. (B) Norepinephrine is the postganglionic mediator.

32. (B) The term for dilation of the pupil is mydriasis.

33. (C) About 46% of all persons have type O blood. Type A is the next most common.

34. (A) Erythropoietin is a glycoprotein that is produced in the kidney and stimulates red blood cell production. It stimulates the division and differentiation of erythroid progenitors in bone marrow. Filgrastim, a human granulocyte colony stimulating factor (G-CSF) regulates the production of neutrophils in the bone marrow. GM-CSF (sargramostim) stimulates granulocytes and macrophages. Oprelvekin is a thrombopoietic growth factor that directly stimulates the proliferation of hematopoietic stem cells and megakaryocytes resulting in platelet production.

35. (D) They transmit impulse to the entire heart.

36. (C) The impulse arises at the SA node.

37. **(D)** Rales are usually associated with disease of the lungs or bronchi.

38. **(D)** Hodgkin's disease involves chronic enlargement of the lymph nodes.

39. **(D)** Phagocytized particles and foreign proteins are filtered out by the lymph glands.

40. **(E)** Diverticulosis is most commonly found in the sigmoid colon after age 40.

41. **(C)** The thalamus is made up of second-order neurons.

42. **(A)** Proton pump inhibitors do not affect cholinergic or histamine H_2 receptors, but suppress gastric acid secretion via specific inhibition of the H^+/K^+ ATPase enzyme system at the secretory surface of the gastric parietal cell. Because the enzyme system is the acid (proton) pump within the gastric mucosa, these drugs are known as pump inhibitors.

43. **(A)** "Hypermetropic" also means a person is far-sighted.

44. **(D)** There is a marked loss of function.

45. **(D)** Micelles are needed to dissolve fatty substances.

46. **(B)** Histoplasmosis usually is caused by *Histoplasma capsulatum,* a soil fungus.

47. **(C)** Potassium is the principal intrinsic ion.

48. **(A)** Interstices are rich in sodium.

49. **(C)** Heavy metals are powerful protein precipitants and create massive imbalance.

50. **(C)** Xerostomia is from the Greek words *xeros,* meaning dry, and *stoma,* meaning mouth.

51. (C) Polycythemia is a type of anemia caused by an excessive number of red blood cells.

52. (C) Bilirubin is the end product of degradation.

53. (B) The ureters are the ducts to the bladder.

54. (B) The gallbladder concentrates bile 10-fold.

55. (D) Crohn's disease is ulcerative colitis.

56. (D) Neutrophils constitute 60% of all white blood cells.

57. (D) ACTH is necessary to trigger or stop secretion.

58. (D) Injury and toxic chemicals also cause acute renal failure, but septicemia is a common cause.

59. (A) Tourette's syndrome, characterized by recurrent non-rhythmic motor or vocal tics, is usually most responsive to dopamine receptor antagonists (e.g., haloperidol) or pimozide.

60. (A) Pyelonephritis usually involves fibrosis and scarring.

61. (A) There is loss of total function and tissue death.

62. (A) Sternum is from the Greek word *sternos,* which means chest.

63. (D) Dyspnea is derived from the Greek words *dys,* meaning bad, and *pnoe,* meaning breathing.

64. (C) The abnormal shape of red blood cells can cause vascular occlusions.

65. (D) A toxic goiter produces symptoms of hyperthyroidism, which is characterized by weight loss, heat intolerance, thinning of the hair, fatigue, and nervousness.

66. (C) During REM, the subject is protected from harm while dreaming by a loss of motor function. The eyes appear to be rapidly moving back and forth. If awakened, the patient describes dreams in great detail.

67. **(B)** Narcolepsy is characterized by sudden sleep attacks.

68. **(A)** Delusional parasitosis is an uncommon disorder in which patients believe that they are infested with insects, typically of the skin, scalp, or ears. Symptoms are persistent, often causing the patient to seek medical attention from a variety of physicians before diagnosis is confirmed. Although a psychiatric referral is warranted in these cases, many patients are extremely resistant to this idea and seek repeated medical attention for skin manifestations (itching, excoriations) from dermatologists and/or general practitioners. Delusional parasitosis occurs more frequently in women than men and typically has an onset in middle age. Evaluation of the true cause of the patient's problem is essential in determining appropriate therapy.

69. **(E)** Each of these findings is indicative of inflammation or damage to the liver. Elevated serum enzyme levels may appear 7–10 days before jaundice.

70. **(A)** Hyperthyroidism produces increased metabolism of all body systems because of the presence of excessive thyroid hormones.

71. **(B)** Raynaud's phenomenon or episodic digital vasoconstriction occurs as a secondary manifestation of many systemic and arterial diseases, including atherosclerosis, thromboangitis obliterans, repeated trauma to the hand, various neurogenic lesions, drug and heavy metal intoxication, or collagen diseases (scleroderma).

72. **(C)** Insulin can produce a wasting of lipoid tissue because of repeated injection at one site. In addition, fat pads can be seen, especially on the thighs, where the patient fails to rotate injection sites.

73. **(A)** The parathyroid secretes a hormone that regulates calcium secretion and tubular reabsorption of phosphate.

74. (D) Intrinsic factor is a glycoprotein of molecular weight 50,000 that is secreted by the gastric mucosal cells.

75. (B) Muscle strength is significantly reduced because of a disorder of neuromuscular function. Smooth muscle is not directly affected.

76. (B) Physical blockage occurs because of swelling of the trabecular network or buildup of debris.

77. (A) In psoriasis, the normal growth regulating control in the skin is lost. A normal turnover time of about 30 days is reduced to 4–5 days, with a resulting accumulation of scales on the surface of the lesion.

78. (E) All of these symptoms are associated with toxic shock syndrome.

79. (E) Inflammation of the conjunctiva may be caused by any of these agents. Redness, burning, and itching of the eye may be accompanied by discharge.

80. (E) The use of immunosuppressive drugs also increases the risk of vaginal candidiasis.

81. (E) A history of renal disease is a significant risk factor for hypertension. Oral decongestants (such as phenylpropranolamine and pseudoephedrine) and fenfluramine are two drug-related causes of increased blood pressure.

82. (D) Cardiac output = stroke volume × heart rate. Decreased cardiac output results in decreased tissue perfusion (especially to the skin and GI tract) with shunting of blood supply to vital organs such as the CNS and myocardium.

83. (C) Decreased coronary blood flow causes an imbalance in myocardial oxygen demand and supply. Abnormal coronary vascular tone and thrombi formation may also cause angina.

84. (E) Vitamin K is essential in the formation of clotting factors II, VII, IX, X, and protein C.

85. **(B)** During an exacerbation of asthma, the small airways become occluded during expiration. There are multiple triggers known to produce bronchospasms in asthmatics.

86. **(C)** Dose-related pulmonary fibrosis is relatively common with amiodarone (Cordarone) and bleomycin (Blenoxane). Aspirin is a known trigger for acute asthma attacks but is not known to cause pulmonary fibrosis.

87. **(D)** Stroke and head injury patients are at high risk for developing aspiration pneumonia. The use of broad spectrum antibiotics suppresses the normal bacterial flora and allows colonization of pathogenic bacteria.

88. **(A)** The use of combination antibiotic therapy for *H pylori* has significantly improved outcome in patients with peptic ulcer disease.

89. **(C)** The normal range for creatinine clearance values is 100–125 mL/min/1.73 m^2.

90. **(D)** Tinea versicolor is a superficial fungal infection that causes a change in skin pigmentation. Topical antifungals may be prescribed.

91. **(E)** The stratum corneum is a semipermeable membrane that acts as a barrier to the passive diffusion of drugs.

92. **(A)** In psoriasis, the average life of epidermal cells is 30–40 hours, versus 300 hours for normal cells.

93. **(E)** The outer layer of the eye is composed of the sclera, a fibrous membrane forming most of the outer envelope; the conjunctiva, a mucous membrane; and the cornea, which forms the anterior sixth of the outer coat and has both lipophilic and hydrophilic layers.

94. **(C)** Most type II (NIDDM) diabetics exhibit insulin tissue resistance possibly mediated by a decreased number of insulin receptors in target cells. Circulating islet cell anti-

bodies are usually negative, only present in less than 10% of NIDDM patients.

95. (C) Potassium deficiency is a well-known cause of cardiac abnormalities. Magnesium plays an important role in maintaining intracellular potassium levels.

6

Clinical Pharmacy

1. Based on Ms. Grant's profile, the penicillin order should be questioned because the
   A. dose is too low
   B. dose is too high
   C. patient is hypokalemic
   D. patient is hyperkalemic
   E. Jarisch–Herxheimer reaction is likely to occur

2. On interviewing Ms. Grant, it is discovered that she has experienced a past allergic reaction to penicillin, which she described as "sudden trouble breathing and a bright red rash." The penicillin order is discontinued immediately. You recommend an alternative antibiotic order of
   A. cefazolin 1 g q 8 h
   B. cefazolin 500 mg q 6 h
   C. ampicillin 1 g q 12 h
   D. erythromycin 500 mg q 6 h
   E. ampicillin/sulbactam 1.5 g q 6 h

3. A normal serum creatinine lab value is
   A. 0.2 mg%
   B. 1.1 mg/dL
   C. 3 mg%
   D. 6 mg/dL
   E. 0.8 mg/L

PATIENT RECORD—ACUTE CARE INSTITUTION

Name:	Dorothy Grant
Address:	Huron Street
Age:	43 yr
Gender:	Female
Weight:	136 lb
Height:	62 inches
Allergies:	Unknown
Patient Complaint:	Flulike symptoms × 5 days, fever
Admitting Diagnosis:	Pneumonia
Past Medical History:	Chronic Glomerulonephritis

LABORATORY DIAGNOSTIC TESTS

Hemoglobin	7.8 g/dL
Hematocrit	31.5%
WBC	16,800 cells/mm^3
Serum Creatinine	3.2 mg/dL
BUN	64 mg/dL
BP	150/98
Na$^+$/K$^+$	145/6.0 mEq/L

ADMISSION ORDERS

Penicillin G Potassium	2 million units IV q 8 h
Amophojel	30 cc PO bid
Captopril	25 mg PO bid
Allopurinol	100 mg PO qd
Calcium carbonate	1 g PO bid

Figure 6–1

4. Many drugs are excreted renally and dosage adjustments are based on estimated creatinine clearance. Ms. Grant's creatinine clearance is estimated using the Cockroft–Gault equation:

$$[140 - \text{age (wt in kg)}/72 \times \text{serum creatinine}] \times 0.85 \text{ (female)}$$

Her creatinine clearance is
A. 160 mL/min
B. 60 mL/min
C. 26 mL/min
D. 22 mL/min
E. 12 mL/min

5. Below what level of creatinine clearance is it necessary to begin adjustment for most renally excreted drugs?
A. 5 mL/min
B. 10 mL/min
C. 50 mL/min
D. 85 mL/min
E. 120 mL/min

6. Two days after admission, the microbiology sputum report identifies a gram-negative organism susceptible to gentamicin, not penicillin. An appropriate gentamicin order would be
A. 7 mg/kg IV q 24 h
B. 100 mg PO q 8 h
C. 1.5 mg/kg IM q 8 h
D. 1.5 mg/kg IV q 36 h
E. 3 mg IV q 8 h

7. The usual serum half-life of gentamicin in adult patients with normal renal function is
A. 2 h
B. 6 h
C. 12 h
D. 18 h
E. 24 h

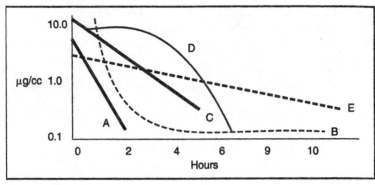

Figure 6–2. Log-plasma concentration curves.

8. Figure 6–2 shows log–plasma concentration curves. The serum concentration–time curve most likely to be observed for gentamicin in Ms. Grant is
   A. A
   B. B
   C. C
   D. D
   E. E

9. Alternative antibiotics that could be prescribed to treat a gram-negative infection include
   I. ciprofloxacin
   II. imipenem
   III. aztreonam

   A. I only
   B. III only
   C. I and II only
   D. II and III only
   E. I, II, and III

10. The purpose of allopurinol therapy in this patient is to
    A. treat nausea and vomiting
    B. inhibit uric acid production
    C. treat hypercalcemia
    D. inhibit gastric acid secretion
    E. treat hypertension

11. An alternative antacid to amphojel suitable for administration to this patient is
    A. Milk of Magnesia
    B. sodium bicarbonate
    C. aluminum hydroxide
    D. Alka-Seltzer
    E. Di-Gel

DIRECTIONS (Questions 12–18): Refer to the patient profile for Laine Edwards (Figure 6–3).

MEDICATION PROFILE—COMMUNITY

Name:	Laine Edwards		
Address:	114 Oakview Avenue		
Age:	72 yr	Gender:	Female
Weight:	97 lb	Height:	5'0"
Allergies:	Sulfa, Codeine		
Smoking history:	None		
Diagnosis:	Primary	Osteoporosis, UTI	
	Secondary	Mild CHF	

MEDICATION RECORD

Date	Rx#	Physician	Drug	Sig	Qty	Ref
2/10	37695	Bailey	Digoxin	0.125 mg PO qd	30	6
2/10	37696	Bailey	HCTZ	25 mg PO qd	30	6
4/07	41984	Bailey	Alendronate	10 mg PO qd	30	6
5/12	42008	Finch	Ciprofloxacin	400 mg PO bid	14	NR

OTC HISTORY

3/18	Centrum Silver 1 tab QD
4/07	Calcium citrate 1 tab (200 mg elemental calcium) TID pc

Figure 6–3

12. Which of Ms. Edwards' drugs is not commercially available in the strength prescribed?
   A. Alendronate
   B. Ciprofloxacin
   C. Calcium citrate
   D. Digoxin
   E. Hydrochlorthiazide

13. Which of Ms. Edwards' medications is most likely to cause a hypersensitivity reaction?
   A. HCTZ
   B. Alendronate
   C. Digoxin
   D. Calcium citrate
   E. Ciprofloxacin

14. Thiazide diuretics exert their effects at the
   I. proximal tubule
   II. nephron
   III. distal portion of the ascending loop of Henle

   A. I only
   B. III only
   C. I and II only
   D. II and III only
   E. I, II, and III

15. The recommended daily intake of elemental calcium for postmenopausal women is
   A. 1–1.5 g
   B. 300–500 mg
   C. 100–200 mg
   D. 600–800 mg
   E. 2–2.5 g

16. Alendronate is useful in the treatment of osteoporosis because it
   I. acts as an estrogen replacement
   II. increases intestinal absorption of calcium
   III. inhibits bone resorption

   A. I only
   B. III only

    C. I and II only
    D. II and III only
    E. I, II, and III

17. When dispensing Alendronate, the pharmacist should advise
    Ms. Edwards to
    I. take with a full glass of water
    II. sit upright for 30 min after ingestion
  III. only take with a full meal

    A. I only
    B. III only
    C. I and II only
    D. II and III only
    E. I, II, and III

18. Over-the-counter (OTC) products that should NOT be taken
    concomitantly with ciprofloxacin include
    I. Magnesium hydroxide
    II. Ferrous sulfate
  III. Calcium citrate

    A. I only
    B. III only
    C. I and II only
    D. II and III only
    E. I, II, and III

DIRECTIONS (Questions 19–31): Refer to the patient profile
for Arthur Crumm (Figure 6–4).

---

19. Available dosage forms for cromolyn include
    I. metered-dose inhaler
    II. nebulized solution
  III. IV solution

    A. I only
    B. III only
    C. I and II only
    D. II and III only
    E. I, II, and III

MEDICATION PROFILE—COMMUNITY

Name:	Arthur M. Crumm
Address:	408 Pond Street
Age:	10 yr
Gender:	Male
Weight:	79 lb
Diagnosis:	Moderate asthma

MEDICATION RECORD

Date	Rx#	Physician	Drug	Sig	Qty	Ref
3/03	34968	C. Pelofsky	Cromolyn Spinhaler	1 cap qid	100	6
4/10	36498	C. Pelofsky	Albuterol Inhaler	2 puffs q 6 h prn & 20–30 min before game	1	6
4/10	36499	C. Pelofsky	Theo-Dur 200 mg	1 tab hs	30	6
5/13	38444	J. Brown	Clarithromycin susp	1 tsp bid		0
5/13	38445	J. Brown	Pseudoephedrine 30 tabs	1 TID prn for congestion	30	0
5/13	36498	C. Pelofsky	Refill			
5/13	36499	C. Pelofsky	Refill			
6/09	40001	C. Pelofsky	Beclomethasone Inhaler	2 puffs qid	1	6
6/09	34698	C. Pelofsky	Refill			
6/09	36499	C. Pelofsky	Refill			

OTC HISTORY

3/18	Flintstone vitamins
4/07	Calcium citrate 1 tab (200 mg elemental calcium) TID pc

Figure 6–4

20. Cromolyn sodium is classified pharmacologically as
   A. an anticholinergic agent
   B. a beta-adrenergic agonist
   C. a serotonin antagonist
   D. a mast cell stabilizer
   E. a methylxanthine

21. Peak-flow meter measurements before treatment in a patient with moderate asthma would most likely reveal a (an)
   A. decreased peak expiratory flow rate (PEFR)
   B. increased PEFR
   C. increased flow rate only after exercise
   D. peak flow rate <50%
   E. peak flow rate >100%

22. The pharmacist should instruct a patient requiring a metered dose inhaler to
   I. shake container before administration
   II. inhale slowly while pressing down on canister
   III. wait 1–3 min between puffs

   A. I only
   B. III only
   C. I and II only
   D. II and III only
   E. I, II, and III

23. In patients using more than one canister of albuterol monthly, pharmacists should caution that
   I. beta-adrenergic agents can be addicting
   II. excessive use may cause tachycardia and/or tremors
   III. a reevaluation by the physician is needed

   A. I only
   B. III only
   C. I and II only
   D. II and III only
   E. I, II, and III

24. Albuterol is useful in patients with asthma because it
  A. is a rapid acting anti-inflammatory agent
  B. reduces airway responsiveness
  C. blocks the late phase of allergic reactions
  D. reverses bronchoconstriction
  E. prevents histamine release

25. Which of the following beta-adrenergic agents is **NOT** short acting?
  A. Pirbuterol
  B. Salmeterol
  C. Terbutaline
  D. Albuterol
  E. None of the above

26. Which of the following could be considered a common trigger of asthma?
  A. Pollen
  B. Medications
  C. Exercise
  D. Upper respiratory infection
  E. All of the above

27. Which of the following would be the most effective drug for preventing exercise-induced asthma?
  A. Leukotriene modifiers
  B. Inhaled corticosteroids
  C. Short-acting beta-2 agonists
  D. Long-acting beta-2 agonists
  E. None of the above

28. The patient should be instructed to rinse their mouth after using which of the following inhalers?
  A. Corticosteroid
  B. Anticholinergic
  C. Short-acting beta-2 agonist
  D. Long-acting beta-2 agonist
  E. All of the above

29. On contacting the physician regarding the clarithromycin prescription, he clarifies that the suspension dose should

approximate a dose of 7.5 mg/kg. The final concentration you dispense is
A. 125 mg/5 mL
B. 125 mg/15 mL
C. 250 mg/5 mL
D. 250 mg/15 mL
E. You dispense capsules because clarithromycin is not available as a suspension.

30. While discussing the dose clarification, the pharmacist should also inform the physician regarding the potential drug interaction between
A. azithromycin and albuterol
B. azithromycin and theophylline
C. clarithromycin and theophylline
D. clarithromycin and ephedrine
E. clarithromycin and cromolyn

31. The generic name of Vanceril is
A. dexamethasone
B. beclomethasone
C. triamcinolone
D. flunisolide
E. hydrocortisone

DIRECTIONS (Questions 32–45): Refer to the patient profile for Virginia Banks (Figure 6–5).

---

32. Non–insulin-dependent diabetes mellitus is characterized by
  I. diminished insulin secretion
  II. insulin resistance in the peripheral tissues
  III. increased risk for vascular disease

A. I only
B. III only
C. I and II only
D. II and III only
E. I, II, and III

MEDICATION PROFILE—COMMUNITY

Name: Virgina Banks
Address: 35 West Shore Rd
Age: 58 yr
Gender: Female
Weight: 182 lb
Diagnosis: Diabetes mellitus, Obesity, Poorly controlled hypertension

MEDICATION RECORD

Date	Rx#	Physician	Drug	Sig	Qty	Ref
3/15	11347	Whitfield	Captopril	12.5 mg tid	90	6
6/15	11347		Refill		90	5
7/07	12496	Whitfield	Acarbose	25 mg in AM	60	2
7/07	12497	Whitfield	HCTZ 50 mg	1 tab daily	60	6
8/06	13877	Zanecchia	Sibutramine	15 mg qd	60	2
8/15	13989	Whitfield	Captopril	25 mg tid	90	6
9/10	12496		Refill			
9/10	12497		Refill			
11/22	14326	Whitfield	Acarbose	50 mg daily	60	1
11/22	14327	Whitfield	Glucotrol 10 mg	1 tab before breakfast	60	1
12/02	14788	Whitfield	Amitriptyline	50 mg qhs	30	1

Figure 6–5

33. The mechanism of action for acarbose involves
    A. stimulation of insulin secretion from pancreas
    B. sensitizing tissue to available insulin
    C. converting insulin from an inactive precursor to its active form
    D. delay of absorption of complex carbohydrates
    E. increasing postprandial insulin concentrations

34. Acarbose must be given at meal times because
   I. food increases bioavailability
   II. acarbose causes diarrhea when taken on an empty stomach
   III. the site of action of acarbose is the small intestines

   A. I only
   B. III only
   C. I and II only
   D. II and III only
   E. I, II, and III

35. Why is sibutramine not a good choice for this patient?
   A. Contraindicated in patients with diabetes
   B. Contraindicated in patients with poorly controlled hypertension
   C. Contraindicated with concurrent MAO inhibitors
   D. Contraindicated with concurrent ACE inhibitors
   E. None of the above

36. Amitriptyline may be prescribed in this patient for which of the following indications?
   A. Seizures
   B. Neuropathy
   C. Stained teeth
   D. A and B
   E. A, B, and C

37. Which of the following sulfonylureas has the longest duration of action?
   A. Acetazolamide
   B. Glyburide
   C. Chlorpropamide
   D. Tolazamide
   E. All are about equal

38. Signs and symptoms of hypoglycemia include
   A. confusion
   B. sweating
   C. headache
   D. weakness
   E. all of the above

39. Possible treatment of hypoglycemia does **NOT** include
   A. insulin
   B. candy
   C. glucose
   D. fruit juice
   E. glucagon

40. Which of the following measures is necessary to prevent the consequences of neuropathy and peripheral vascular decline in diabetic patients?
   A. Weekly inspection of skin
   B. Use of tightly fitted shoes
   C. Discouragement of self-treatment of warts, corns, and calluses
   D. Routine anaerobic exercise
   E. Avoid use of elasticized support stockings

41. Which of the following is (are) symptomatic of ketoacidosis?
   A. Perspiration
   B. Dry skin
   C. Acetone breath
   D. Excitation
   E. B and C

42. In hyperglycemic coma, blood glucose levels can reach
   A. 200 µg/dL
   B. 300 µg/dL
   C. 50 µg/dL
   D. 800 µg/dL
   E. 200 g/dL

43. Which of the following may be observed in patients with diabetic neuropathy?
   A. Incontinence
   B. Gastric atony
   C. Diarrhea
   D. Impotence
   E. All of the above

44. When Mrs. Banks's blood pressure medication was changed from HCTZ to propranolol, she became at risk for
   A. hypercalcemia
   B. hypokalemia
   C. hyperlipidemia
   D. hyperglycemia
   E. hypoglycemia

45. Which of the following antihypertensive agents has **NO** adverse effect on glucose tolerance?
   I. Metoprolol
   II. Atenolol
   III. Captopril

   A. I only
   B. III only
   C. I and II only
   D. II and III only
   E. I, II, and III

DIRECTIONS (Questions 46–57): Refer to the patient profile for Sandra Mathers (Figure 6–6).

---

46. Ortho-Novum 777 is classified as what type of contraceptive?
   I. Monophasic
   II. Biphasic
   III. Triphasic

   A. I only
   B. III only
   C. I and II only
   D. II and III only
   E. I, II, and III

MEDICATION PROFILE—COMMUNITY

Name: Sandra Mathers
Address: 14 Reservoir Avenue
Age: 28 yr
Gender: Female
Allergies: Aspirin

MEDICATION RECORD

Date	Rx#	Physician	Drug	Sig	Qty		Ref
1/11/00	4421	Peters	Amoxicillin 500 mg	1 cap tid	30		0
3/10/00	6710	Peters	Ortho-Novum 777	1 tab qd	28	Dial-pak	12
7/10/00	7112	Smith	Tetracycline 250 mg	1 cap qid	60		5
10/10/01	7882	Jenkins	Nystatin vaginal tabs	1 qhs	15		0
2/15/02	8990	Jenkins	Prenatal vitamins	1 tab qd	100		3

Figure 6–6

47. When dispensing the Ortho-Novum for the first time, the pharmacist should counsel the patient
   I. that oral contraceptives do not protect against HIV or other sexually transmitted diseases
   II. to take 1 tablet daily at the same time each day if possible
   III. to read the accompanying patient information insert

   A. I only
   B. III only
   C. I and II only
   D. II and III only
   E. I, II, and III

48. In April 2001, Ms. Mathers contacts you because she forgot to take her birth control pill yesterday. Which of the following instructions is correct?
   A. Take 2 tablets today and continue with cycle
   B. Take 2 tablets for the next 3 days

C. Use an additional form of contraception for the remainder of the cycle

D. A and C

E. B and C

49. In July, Ms. Mathers indicates that her tetracycline prescription is for a recurrent adult acne problem. What advice would you provide when counseling her about this prescription?

A. Avoid prolonged exposure to sunlight

B. Avoid simultaneous ingestion with dairy products

C. Recommend an alternative or additional form of contraception

D. A and B

E. A, B, and C

50. What extra labels should be included on the nystatin prescription?

I. Do not take by mouth

II. Do not crush

III. Avoid caffeinated beverages while taking this medication

A. I only

B. III only

C. I and II only

D. II and III only

E. I, II, and III

51. Which of Ms. Mathers' medications may be responsible for her yeast infection in October?

A. Oral contraceptives

B. Tetracycline

C. Amoxicillin

D. A and B

E. A and C

52. What counseling should the pharmacist provide when Ms. Mathers presents the prenatal vitamin prescription?
    A. Confirm that use of the Ortho-Novum prescription has been discontinued
    B. Keep the vitamins refrigerated in original container
    C. Take the vitamin with dairy products to avoid stomach upset
    D. Provide a list of alcohol-free over-the-counter products
    E. Suggest the use of supplemental contraceptives while taking vitamins

53. In April 2001, Ms. Mathers visited your pharmacy complaining of a headache. What product(s) should **NOT** be recommended?
    I. Bayer Plus
    II. Ascriptin
    III. Excedrin

    A. I only
    B. III only
    C. I and II only
    D. II and III only
    E. I, II, and III

54. In May 2002, the patient developed a urinary tract infection. Which is the most appropriate antibiotic for treatment?
    A. Trimethoprim–sulfamethoxazole
    B. Penicillin
    C. Tetracycline
    D. Vancomycin
    E. Ciprofloxacin

55. In June 2002, Ms. Mathers revisits your pharmacy complaining of mild to moderate stomach upset. Which of the following products would you recommend?
    I. Metoclopramide
    II. Nizatidine
    III. Maalox

    A. I only
    B. III only

  C. I and II only
  D. II and III only
  E. I, II, and III

56. One month after Ms. Mathers had her baby she has complaints of exacerbated allergy symptoms. She plans to nurse her infant for at least 6 months. Which of the following nonprescription products would you recommend?
  A. Diphenhydramine
  B. Clemastine
  C. Pyrilamine
  D. Chlorpheniramine
  E. None of the above

57. How early can oral contraceptives be restarted postpartum in a nonnursing mother?
  A. 1–2 weeks
  B. 2–4 weeks
  C. 4–6 weeks
  D. 6–8 weeks
  E. 8–10 weeks

DIRECTIONS (Questions 58–67): Refer to the patient profile for Jessica Whitfield (Figure 6–7).

---

58. A possible indication for the use of ibuprofen in this patient is
  I. rheumatoid arthritis
  II. dysmenorrhea
  III. fever reduction

  A. I only
  B. III only
  C. I and II only
  D. II and III only
  E. I, II, and III

PATIENT PRESCRIPTION		
Jessica Whitfield		12909 Delmar St
Rx:	Ibuprofen 800 mg	
	Dispense #120	
Sig:	1 tab qid	Refill: 3

Figure 6–7

59. Which of the following auxiliary labels should be placed on the medicine container?

A. Keep refrigerated
B. Protect from light and heat
C. Take with food and milk
D. Take at least 1 h before meals
E. None of the above

60. The primary mechanism of action of ibuprofen is inhibition of prostaglandin synthesis. Prostaglandins

A. inhibit gastric acid secretion
B. stimulate uterine contractions
C. reduce inflammation
D. A and B only
E. do all of the above

61. Ms. Whitfield visits your pharmacy in July 2001 with complaints of chronic stomach upset. Which of the following products would you recommend?

A. Magnesium hydroxide
B. Aluminum hydroxide
C. Famotidine
D. Cimetidine
E. None of the above; refer to physician

62. After a visit to her physician and evaluation for peptic ulceration, Ms. Whitfield visits your pharmacy with a prescription for misoprostol 200 μg qid. Which of the following labels should be placed on the medication container?

A. Keep refrigerated
B. Protect from light and heat

   C. Take with food

   D. Take at least 1 hour before meals

   E. None of the above

63. What is the most likely indication for the misoprostol in this patient?

   A. Prevention of NSAID gastric ulcer

   B. Improvement of renal function

   C. Rheumatoid arthritis

   D. Prevention of NSAID urinary crystallization

   E. None of the above

64. What type of drug is misoprostol?

   A. Histamine-1 antagonist

   B. Histamine-2 antagonist

   C. Prostaglandin

   D. Anticholinergic

   E. Beta-1 agonist

65. When counseling Ms. Whitfield regarding misoprostol, which of the following side effects will she most likely experience?

   A. Diarrhea

   B. Headache

   C. Dysmenorrhea

   D. Cramps

   E. Constipation

66. Which of the following issues would you counsel about Ms. Whitfield regarding the use of misoprostol?

   I. Begin therapy only on second or third day of next normal menstrual period

   II. Ensure compliance with contraceptive measures

   III. Confirm negative serum pregnancy test

   A. I only

   B. III only

   C. I and II only

   D. II and III only

   E. I, II, and III

67. How long should the misoprostol regimen be continued?
   A. 7 days
   B. 14 days
   C. 21 days
   D. 28 days
   E. Continued for the length of NSAID therapy

DIRECTIONS (Questions 68–82): Refer to the patient profile for Jenny Swift (Figure 6–8).

---

68. Which of the drugs prescribed on January 13 would interact with ciprofloxacin?
   I. Magnesium hydroxide
   II. Sucralfate
   III. Ranitidine

   A. I only
   B. III only
   C. I and II only
   D. II and III only
   E. I, II, and III

69. In which of the following ways can smoking affect peptic ulcer disease?
   A. Reduces GI mucosal production of prostaglandins
   B. Delays the healing of ulcers
   C. Reduces GI mucosal blood flow
   D. Increases reflex of duodenal contents into the stomach
   E. All of the above

70. Which of the following pain episodes is typical of duodenal ulcers?
   I. Midepigastric gnawing or burning sensation
   II. Night awakening episode
   III. Pain relieved by food

   A. I only
   B. III only
   C. I and II only
   D. II and III only
   E. I, II, and III

MEDICATION PROFILE—COMMUNITY

Name: Jenny Swift
Address: 1003 Cedar Creek Lane
Age: 49 yr
Gender: Female
Allergies: Tetracycline, Sulfonamides
Diagnosis: Primary: Peptic ulcer
             Secondary: Esophageal reflux
                         Urinary tract infection (1/6/01)
                         Acute lower back pain (4/10/01)
                         Depression (5/10/01)

MEDICATION RECORD

Date	Rx#	Physician	Drug	Sig	Qty	Ref
1/6/01	334	Herrin	Ciprofloxacin 500 mg	500 mg bid	20	0
1/13/01	421	Payne	Magnesium hydroxide liquid	15 mL pc & hs	1 pint	prn
1/13/01	710	Payne	Ranitidine	150 mg bid	60	3
1/13/01	723	Payne	Sucralfate	1 gram qid	100	3
3/13/01	739	Payne	Ranitidine/Bismuth citrate	1 cap bid	56	0
3/13/01	740	Payne	Clarithromycin 500 mg	1 tab tid	42	0
3/20/01	790	Benson	Fexofenadine	160 mg bid	60	3
4/1/01	830	Wilson	Celecoxib	100 mg bid	30	0
5/10/01	900	Smith	Citalopram	20 mg qd	30	4

Figure 6–8

71. The mechanism(s) for antacid therapy in the treatment of peptic ulcers includes

    I. neutralization of gastric acid

    II. inhibition conversion of pepsinogen to pepsin

    III. histamine-2 receptor antagonism

    A. I only

    B. III only

    C. I and II only

    D. II and III only

    E. I, II, and III

72. Histamine-2 receptor antagonists promote healing of ulcers by

    I. neutralizing gastric acid

    II. inhibiting conversion of pepsinogen to pepsin

    III. inhibiting gastric acid secretion via parietal cells

    A. I only

    B. III only

    C. I and II only

    D. II and III only

    E. I, II, and III

73. Sucralfate promotes healing of duodenal ulcers by

    A. neutralizing gastric acid

    B. inhibiting conversion of pepsinogen to pepsin

    C. inhibiting gastric acid secretion via parietal cells

    D. binding to defective GI mucosa (protectant)

    E. none of the above

74. Which of the following foods may exacerbate esophageal reflux?

    A. Coffee

    B. Spicy foods

    C. Peppermint

    D. Processed meats

    E. All of the above

75. Bleeding from a peptic ulcer may be manifested as
    I. coffee-ground vomit
   II. black tarry stools
 III. epistaxis

   A. I only
   B. III only
   C. I and II only
   D. II and III only
   E. I, II, and III

76. What is the most likely reason for prescribing clarithromycin in this patient?
   A. Urinary tract infection
   B. Sinus infection
   C. *Helicobacter pylori* infection
   D. *Escherichia coli* infection
   E. None of the above

77. In which class of drugs is clarithromycin?
   A. Aminoglycosides
   B. Cephalosporins
   C. Tetracyclines
   D. Macrolide antibiotics
   E. None of the above

78. Which of the following prescriptions requires pharmacist intervention to prevent a medication error?
    I. Sucralfate
   II. Ranitidine
 III. Fexofenadine

   A. I only
   B. III only
   C. I and II only
   D. II and III only
   E. I, II, and III

79. Which of the following would be acceptable reasons to NOT dispense the celecoxib to this patient?
  I. Celecoxib is contraindicated for use in patients with active ulcer disease
  II. Celecoxib should not be used in patients with a history of allergies to sulfonamides
  III. Celecoxib should not be used in patients with a history of allergies to tetracyclines

  A. I only
  B. III only
  C. I and II only
  D. II and III only
  E. I, II, and III

80. Which of the following are approved indications for celecoxib?
  I. Acute pain syndromes
  II. Osteoarthritis pain
  III. Familial adenomatous polyposis

  A. I only
  B. III only
  C. I and II only
  D. II and III only
  E. I, II, and III

81. Which of the following analgesics would be appropriate for use in this patient?
  A. Aspirin
  B. Acetaminophen
  C. Rofecoxib
  D. Indomethacin
  E. None of the above

82. Which brand name product would be dispensed for the treatment of depression?
  A. Prozac
  B. Celexa
  C. Sarafem
  D. Celebrex
  E. Zoloft

PATIENT PRESCRIPTION	
Marie Curusio	4905 West 132nd Street
Rx: Fluoxetine	20 mg
Dispense #60	
Sig: 1 Tab qd for ten days each month for PMDD	Refill: 3

Figure 6–9

DIRECTIONS (Questions 83–87): Refer to the patient profile for Maria Curusio (Figure 6–9).

---

83. PMDD is an abbreviation for which of the following terms?
   A. Primary mental depressive disorder
   B. Premenstrual dysphoric disorder
   C. Primary misuse of diuretics disorder
   D. Premenstrual dietary disorder
   E. None of the above

84. Which brand name product would be dispensed for this patient?
   A. Prozac
   B. Sarafem
   C. Celexa
   D. Zoloft
   E. None of the above

85. Which of the following are appropriate dosage regimens for fluoxetine in this patient?
   I. 20 mg/d
   II. 120 mg/d in divided doses
   III. 20 mg/d for 10 days each month

   A. I only
   B. III only
   C. I and II only
   D. II and III only
   E. I, II, and III

86. When Mrs. Curusio picks up her prescription product she also wants to purchase a cough and cold product. Which common ingredient in OTC cough and cold products could result in a drug–drug interaction?

A. Codeine

B. Dextromethorphan

C. Diphenhydramine

D. Guaifenesin

E. None of the above

87. Two months later, Mrs. Curusio is also prescribed sibutramine for weight loss. Which of the following problems might occur during concurrent therapy with her existing regimen?

A. Serotonin syndrome

B. Exacerbation of PMDD

C. Hyperprolactinemia

D. Drowsiness

E. None of the above

DIRECTIONS (Questions 88–105): Refer to the patient profile for Flora Colella (Figure 6–10).

---

88. Phenytoin chewable tablets contain what percentage of phenytoin?

A. 50%

B. 60%

C. 75%

D. 92%

E. 100%

89. Without a loading dose, the maximal anticonvulsant effect after the initiation of phenytoin therapy may be anticipated to occur

A. after the first dose

B. within 24 hours

C. within 48 hours

D. in approximately 1–3 weeks

E. in approximately 6 months

MEDICATION PROFILE—COMMUNITY

Name:	Flora Colella
Address:	220 Baldwin Court
Age:	54 yr
Gender:	Female
Allergies:	None
Diagnosis:	Seizure disorder

MEDICATION RECORD

Date	Rx#	Physician	Drug	Sig	Qty	Ref
1/1	5421	Peters	Phenytoin 50 mg	1 tab tid	100	12
3/10	6711	Peters	Phenytoin 50 mg	1 tab AM, Noon, hs	100	6
7/10	8112	Peters	Dilantin Kapseals 100 mg	1 cap bid	100	6
10/10	7872	Peters	Carbamazepine 100 mg	1 tab tid	50	0
11/12	7923	Peters	Carbamazepine 100 mg chewable tabs	1 tab tid	100	3
12/15	8902	Peters	Dilantin Kapseals 100 mg	1 tab tid	100	6

Figure 6–10

90. Which of the following are common side effects associated with phenytoin therapy?
    I. Nystagmus
    II. Ataxia
    III. Gingival hyperplasia

    A. I only
    B. III only
    C. I and II only
    D. II and III only
    E. I, II, and III

91. What is the most likely reason that the physician specified Dilantin Kapseals?
   A. Kapseals are easier to swallow than other dosage forms
   B. Kapseals may be crushed and given with orange juice
   C. Slow absorption of Kapseals allows for longer dosing interval
   D. Kapseals are the only adult formulation containing 100% phenytoin
   E. None of the above

92. What patient recommendations should the pharmacist make when dispensing carbamazepine?
   I. Take 2 hours before meals
   II. Take with food
   III. May cause drowsiness

   A. I only
   B. III only
   C. I and II only
   D. II and III only
   E. I, II, and III

93. What laboratory test should be monitored with the addition of carbamazepine to her regimen?
   A. Serum uric acid levels
   B. Complete blood counts
   C. Blood glucose levels
   D. All of the above
   E. None of the above

94. In November, Flora is brought into the emergency room with status epilepticus. This term refers to
   A. a sudden loss of balance and lack of eye balance
   B. an outburst of violence or hallucinations
   C. generalized tonic–clonic seizures with no recovery of consciousness between attacks
   D. postictal confusion and muscle flaccidity
   E. sudden repetitive, nonpurposeful movements

95. The drug of choice in status epilepticus is
   A. carbamazepine 600 mg PO
   B. phenytoin 50 mg IM

    C. phenobarbital 600 mg IM
    D. diazepam 10 mg IV
    E. diazepam 0.5 mg IV

96. Once stabilized, Flora is admitted to the hospital. During her stay she received parenteral fosphenytoin. Fosphenytoin is
    A. a prodrug of phenytoin
    B. a metabolite of phenytoin
    C. the levo isomer of phenytoin
    D. the dextro isomer of phenytoin
    E. none of the above

97. Fosphenytoin is monitored by following
    A. plasma phenytoin concentrations
    B. unbound phenytoin concentrations
    C. plasma fosphenytoin concentrations
    D. unbound fosphenytoin concentrations
    E. none of the above

98. Once steady-state concentrations were achieved, Flora's phenytoin level was 15 μg/mL. This serum level indicates
    A. a toxic level; the dosage should be reduced
    B. a level below therapeutic range; the dosage should be increased
    C. a level within therapeutic range
    D. a level at the upper limit of the therapeutic range
    E. none of the above

99. Fosphenytoin amounts and concentrations are expressed in
    A. micrograms
    B. grams
    C. PE units
    D. milliunits
    E. none of the above

100. What is the most likely reason for the increase in phenytoin dosage with the prescription on December 15?
    A. Carbamazepine increased the bioavailability of phenytoin
    B. Carbamazepine induced the metabolism of phenytoin
    C. Carbamazepine enhanced the renal excretion of phenytoin
    D. The patient began to experience absence seizures
    E. The patient was noncompliant

101. Which of the following drugs may increase phenytoin activity?
  A. Salicylates
  B. Omeprazole
  C. Cimetidine
  D. Phenylpropanolamine
  E. A, B, and C

102. Which antibiotic should be avoided in this patient, if possible?
  A. Amoxicillin
  B. Cephalexin
  C. Cefaclor
  D. Penicillin
  E. Erythromycin

103. Dr. Peters is considering adding phenobarbital to Ms. Colella's regimen. Which of the following best describes the mechanism of action of barbiturates in controlling seizures?
  A. Inhibit monosynaptic and polysynaptic transmission and raise seizure threshold in cortex
  B. Stabilize neuronal membranes
  C. Affect limbic system and thalamus
  D. Limit carbonic anhydrase in CNS
  E. Enhance brain concentrations of GABA

104. Therapeutic serum concentrations of phenobarbital for seizure control range from
  A. 60–100 µg/mL
  B. 15–35 µg/mL
  C. 0.01–0.008 µg/mL
  D. 40–80 µg/mL
  E. 2–5 µg/mL

105. Phenobarbital is a known enzyme inducer. This means
  A. phenobarbital is able to inactivate other drugs in a method similar to hepatic enzymes
  B. phenobarbital increases the synthesis of certain enzymes in the liver
  C. adding phenobarbital to a patient's drug regimen increases plasma drug concentrations
  D. all of the above
  E. none of the above

DIRECTIONS (Questions 106–117): Refer to patient profile for Matthew Ryan (Figure 6–11).

106. In parenteral nutrition solutions, the primary source of energy is
A. protein
B. amino acids
C. lipid emulsion
D. carbohydrate
E. vitamins

107. One liter of 10% dextrose contains how much dextrose?
A. 1 g
B. 10 g
C. 100 g
D. 10 mg
E. 100 mg

108. The highest concentration of lipid emulsion that should be infused in a central or peripheral vein is
A. 5%
B. 10%
C. 15%
D. 20%
E. 30%

109. Which of the following statements concerning peripheral parenteral nutrition is FALSE?
A. A peripheral site is recommended if a patient is expected to require parenteral nutrition for <1 week
B. Up to 20% dextrose can be administered peripherally without damaging the vein
C. Up to 20% lipid emulsion can be administered peripherally without damaging the vein
D. Peripheral administration of parenteral nutrition has a lower risk of infection than with central administration
E. A fluid-restricted patient is not a good candidate for peripheral parenteral nutrition

MEDICATION PROFILE—
ACUTE CARE INSTITUTION

Name:	Matthew Ryan
Address:	26251 W. Cedar Niles Circle
Age:	18 yr
Gender:	Male
Weight:	120 lb
Height:	67″
Allergies:	No known drug allergies
Patient Complaint:	Diarrhea, abdominal pain
Diagnosis:	Crohn's disease

LABORATORY DIAGNOSTIC TESTS

Total protein	6.5 gm/dL
Albumin	3.4 gm/dL
Calcium	8.9 gm/dL
Phosphate	2.7 mg/dL
Sodium	140 mEq/L
Potassium	4.0 mEq/L
Chloride	96 mEq/L
Blood glucose	88 mg/dL
Serum creatinine	1.0 mg/dL
BUN	18 mg/dL

ADMISSION ORDERS

Hydrocortisone	100 mg IV q 8 hr
TPN	2.5 L/day Compression schedule

Figure 6–11

110. Which of the following combinations of additives can form an insoluble precipitate and cause potentially life-threatening consequences?
   A. Sodium and calcium
   B. Potassium and calcium
   C. Phosphorus and calcium
   D. Magnesium and phosphorus
   E. Potassium and magnesium

111. Which of the following factors influence calcium and phosphate incompatibility?
   A. Concentration
   B. pH
   C. Temperature
   D. Time
   E. All of the above

112. Which of the following calculations is false?
   A. 1 g protein yields 4 kcal/kg
   B. 1 g fat yields 9 kcal/g
   C. 1 g yields 3.4 kcal/g
   D. lipid emulsion 10% provides 1.1 cal/mL
   E. None are false

113. Which of the following drugs is used to treat refractory Crohn's disease?
   A. Methotrexate
   B. Infliximab
   C. Allopurinol
   D. Lopressor
   E. Ranitidine

114. In addition to Crohn's disease, infliximab is also indicated for the treatment of
   I. rheumatoid arthritis
   II. pancreatitis
   III. osteoarthritis

   A. I only
   B. II only
   C. I and II only
   D. II and III only
   E. I, II, and III

115. Infliximab is administered via
- **A.** rectal enema
- **B.** oral solution
- **C.** rectal suppositories
- **D.** IV infusion
- **E.** subcutaneous infusion

116. Which of the following side effects have been associated with infliximab use?
- **A.** Tuberculosis
- **B.** Sepsis
- **C.** Histoplasmosis
- **D.** A and B
- **E.** A, B, and C

117. Because of the increased risk of infection, which of the following agents should not be administered concurrently with infliximab?
- **I.** Live vaccines
- **II.** Acetaminophen
- **III.** Sumtatriptan

- **A.** I only
- **B.** II only
- **C.** I and II
- **D.** II and III
- **E.** I, II, and III

DIRECTIONS (Questions 118–122): Refer to the following prescription.

PATIENT PRESCRIPTION		
Tara Bryan	Age: 2 yr	Weight: 26 lb
Dx: Acute otitis media		
Rx: Amoxicillin/clavulanate 250 mg/5 mL		150 mL
Sig: 1 tsp TID × 10 days	Refill: NR	

118. Signs and symptoms of acute otitis media do **NOT** include
   A. fever
   B. irritability
   C. stiff neck
   D. lethargy
   E. the child may be asymptomatic

119. The purpose of the addition of clavulanic acid to amoxicillin is to
   I. decrease the incidence of diarrhea
   II. increase palatability
   III. expand bacterial coverage

   A. I only
   B. III only
   C. I and II only
   D. II and III only
   E. I, II, and III

120. Alternative antibiotics for otitis media for the child allergic to penicillin include all of the following **EXCEPT**
   A. clindamycin
   B. erythromycin
   C. erythromycin–sulfisoxazole
   D. ciprofloxacin
   E. trimethropin–sulfamethoxazole

121. When dispensing the prescription, the pharmacist should counsel Tara's caregiver
   I. to keep the medication refrigerated
   II. the medication may cause diarrhea or loose stools
   III. to give 1 hour before meals on an empty stomach

   A. I only
   B. III only
   C. I and II
   D. II and III
   E. I, II, and III

122. Two weeks after having the prescription filled, Tara's mother returns to the pharmacy and complains that Tara's symptoms are back. Possible explanation(s) include

   I. treatment failure due to noncompliance
  II. resistant organism
 III. reinfection

  A. I only
  B. III only
  C. I and II
  D. II and III
  E. I, II, and III

DIRECTIONS (Questions 123–127): Refer to the following prescription.

PATIENT PRESCRIPTION

Maria Romano   Age: 31 yr   Weight: 72 kg
Dx: Hashimoto's thyroiditis
Rx: Liotrix 1/2 grain   30 tabs
Sig: 1 tab QD   Refill: 3

123. Hashimoto's thyroiditis can be described as
  A. an infection of the thyroid gland
  B. toxic diffuse goiter
  C. another name for Graves' disease
  D. a common cause of hypothyroidism
  E. result of a pituitary adenoma

124. Liotrix contains
  A. thyroxine (T_4) only
  B. triiodothyronine (T_3) only
  C. 2:1 ratio of T_4:T_3
  D. 4:1 ratio of T_3:T_4
  E. 4:1 ratio of T_4:T_3

125. Maximal effects from Liotrix therapy would be anticipated in
  A. 24 hours
  B. 48 hours
  C. 72 hours
  D. 1 week
  E. 1 month

126. Desiccated thyroid **CANNOT** be substituted for Liotrix because
  I. it contains only T_4
  II. it is available only in 2-, 3-, and 5-grain strengths
  III. potency is variable because it is standardized by iodine content

  A. I only
  B. III only
  C. I and II
  D. II and III
  E. I, II, and III

127. Levothyroxine (synthetic T_4) is a recommended thyroid replacement preparation for patients with Hashimoto's thyroiditis because
  A. the body does not require T_3 for thyroid function
  B. T_4 is 10 times more potent than T_3
  C. T_4 is metabolized to T_3 in the periphery
  D. T_4 is not inactivated by proteins
  E. there are no reported drug interactions with T_4

DIRECTIONS (Questions 128–140): Refer to patient profile for Jamie Brown (Figure 6–12).

128. Which of the following is (are) classic sign(s) of type 1 diabetes?
  A. Polydipsia
  B. Weight gain
  C. Polyuria
  D. Fatigue
  E. A, C, and D

MEDICATION PROFILE—COMMUNITY

Name:	Jamie Brown
Address:	77 Bleek Street
Age:	75 yr
Weight:	74.4 kg
Gender:	Female
Allergies:	None
Diagnosis:	Type I Diabetes mellitus

MEDICATION RECORD

Date	Rx#	Physician	Drug	Sig	Qty	Ref
3/2	67493	Luis	Humulin Reg 100 u	30 u qAM	10 cc	12
	67494	Luis	Humulin Lente 100 u	20 u qAM & hs	10 cc	12
	67495	Luis	Insulin syringes 27 g	ut dict	100	prn
	67496	Luis	Nystatin vaginal cream	use AM & PM	tube	11
4/1	67493		Refill		10 cc	11
	67494		Refill		10 cc	11

Figure 6–12

129. Which of the following values is indicative of diabetes mellitus?
    A. Fasting blood glucose of 140 mg/dL or more
    B. Blood glucose level of 200 mg/dL 2 hours postprandial
    C. Random blood glucose of 200 mg/dL
    D. A and B
    E. A, B, and C

130. Diabetics should eat a well-balanced diet that includes what percentage of complex carbohydrates on a daily basis?
    A. 55–65%
    B. 10–15%
    C. 30–35%
    D. 5–10%
    E. 75–90%

131. Humulin insulin is derived from
   A. human donors
   B. beef
   C. enzymatic cleavage of porcine insulin
   D. recombinant DNA technology
   E. filtration of bovine insulin

132. Lente insulin is classified as
   A. a zinc–insulin mixture
   B. a mixture of 30% ultralente and 70% regular insulin
   C. a long-acting insulin
   D. an intermediate-acting insulin
   E. A and D

133. A typical total daily insulin dose for a type 1 diabetic adult patient is
   A. 0.5–1.0 u/kg
   B. 0.1–0.5 u/kg
   C. 1.5–3.0 u/kg
   D. 3.0–5.0 u/kg
   E. not based on patient weight

134. Insulin syringes for U-100 insulins are available in all the following sizes **EXCEPT**
   A. 1/100 cc
   B. 1/4 cc
   C. 3/10 cc
   D. 1/2 cc
   E. 1 cc

135. Instructions for the patient for handling and storage of her insulin include
   I. store in a cool place; do not freeze
   II. do not use the regular insulin if cloudy
   III. shake or rotate the lente insulin so that it appears uniformly cloudy prior to injection

   A. I only
   B. III only
   C. I and II
   D. II and III
   E. I, II, and III

136. Which of the following can precipitate diabetic ketoacidosis?
   A. Exercise
   B. Infection
   C. Stress
   D. Dietary noncompliance
   E. All of the above

137. Symptoms of diabetic coma include
   A. dehydration
   B. hypotension
   C. nausea and vomiting
   D. polydipsia
   E. all of the above

138. Therapy for hyperglycemic coma involves
   A. IV glucose
   B. regular insulin
   C. fluids
   D. electrolyte reduction
   E. B and C

139. Which of the following is **NOT** observed as a complication of diabetes?
   A. Gastroparesis
   B. Nephropathy
   C. Hypotension
   D. Blindness
   E. Peripheral neuropathy

140. To correct excessive preprandial glucose concentrations, patients should use supplemental doses of
   A. regular insulin
   B. NPH insulin
   C. lente insulin
   D. ultralente insulin
   E. a mixture of regular and NPH insulin

DIRECTIONS (Questions 141–143): Refer to the following acute care case:

The emergency department calls the pharmacy regarding a 28-year-old male patient who is suspected of having methanol poisoning. The patient is seizing, has a pulse rate of 104 beats/min, and a respiratory rate of 48 breaths/min. The physician plans to treat the methanol poisoning with IV ethanol using the recommended 10% v/v alcohol solution. On hand in the pharmacy is 5% v/v alcohol and 95% v/v alcohol.

141. The recommended treatment for seizures when a rapid response is required is
    A. phenytoin 1 g IV push
    B. phenytoin 200 mg IM
    C. phenobarbital 60 mg IV push
    D. diazepam 5 mg IV over 2–3 min
    E. midazolam 20 mg IV

142. Ethanol is administered in methanol poisonings because it
    I. corrects the metabolic alkalosis
    II. hastens the renal excretion of methanol
    III. prevents the formation of formic acid

    A. I only
    B. III only
    C. I and II
    D. II and III
    E. I, II, and III

143. How much 95% v/v and 5% v/v alcohol are needed to make 1 L of 10% v/v alcohol?
    A. 95%–42 mL, 5%–958 mL
    B. 95%–56 mL, 5%–944 mL
    C. 95%–68 mL, 5%–932 mL
    D. 95%–112 mL, 5%–888 mL
    E. 95%–130 mL, 5%–870 mL

DIRECTIONS (Questions 144–152): Refer to the community profile for Karen Howland (Figure 6–13).

144. Lithium carbonate is classified as an
  I. antimanic
  II. antidepressant
  III. mood stabilizer

  A. I only
  B. III only
  C. I and II
  D. II and III
  E. I, II, and III

MEDICATION PROFILE—COMMUNITY

Name: Karen Howland
Address: 132 Ninety Avenue
Age: 36 yr
Weight: 104 lb
Gender: Female
Allergies: None
Diagnosis: Bipolar depression, atypical depression

MEDICATION RECORD

Date	Rx#	Physician	Drug	Sig	Qty	Ref
10/19	5891	Fried	Lithium carbonate 300 mg	2 caps qAM & hs	100	2
	5892	Fried	Valproic acid 250 mg	2 caps qAM & hs	100	NR
11/17	5891		Refill		100	1
	7043	Fried	Valproic acid 250 mg	2 caps tid	200	2
	7044	Fried	Fluoxetine 20 mg	1 qid	30	3

Figure 6–13

145. Lithium therapy should be withheld if the patient's serum concentration exceeds
   A. 0.5 mEq/L
   B. 1.0 mg/L
   C. 2.0 mEq/L
   D. 5.0 mg/mL
   E. 7.0 mEq/L

146. It is important that the patient recognizes all the following signs as possible lithium side effects **EXCEPT**
   A. hand tremors
   B. headaches
   C. muscle weakness
   D. constipation
   E. polyuria

147. When dispensing the lithium prescription, the pharmacist should counsel the patient to
   I. avoid dehydration
   II. be aware of impaired mental alertness
   III. take with meals

   A. I only
   B. III only
   C. I and II
   D. II and III
   E. I, II, and III

148. Optimal response to a lithium dosage regimen is usually observed in
   A. 14 days
   B. 7 days
   C. 48 h
   D. 24 h
   E. 6 h

149. Valproic acid is also indicated in the treatment of
   A. anxiety attacks
   B. absence seizures
   C. tonic–clonic seizures
   D. obsessive–compulsive disorder
   E. status epilepticus

150. The generic name for Prozac is
  A. fluoxetine
  B. sertraline
  C. paroxetine
  D. trazodone
  E. imipramine

151. The addition of fluoxetine to the current medication regimen may
  A. decrease lithium requirements
  B. increase serum valproic acid levels
  C. induce valproic acid metabolism
  D. reduce insomnia
  E. minimize tremors

152. The patient asks the pharmacist's advice about a nonprescription drug to treat heartburn. The pharmacist advises her that any of the following are acceptable **EXCEPT**
  A. famotidine
  B. nizatidine
  C. cimetidine
  D. ranitidine
  E. aluminum hydroxide

DIRECTIONS (Questions 153–167): Refer to the patient profile for Jonathan Whitfield (Figure 6–14).

---

153. The purpose of the digoxin orders on March 20 in this patient is to
  I. achieve rapid digitalization
  II. increase cardiac output
  III. achieve a digoxin serum level above 2.0 ng/mL

  A. I only
  B. III only
  C. I and II only
  D. II and III only
  E. I, II, and III

MEDICATION PROFILE—INSTITUTION

Name: Jonathan Whitfield
Address: 4905 West 133rd Terrace
Age: 57 yr
Weight: 200 lb
Height: 5'11"
Gender: Male
Allergies: None
Diagnosis: CHF, Ascites, Pedal edema

LABORATORY TESTS

3/20	Serum sodium	130
	Serum potassium	3.5
	Creatinine	1.0
	Blood pressure	120/70
	Pulse	100
3/22	Serum digoxin	1.2 ng/mL

MEDICATION ORDERS

Date	Drug/Strength	Route	Sig
3/20	Digoxin 0.5 mg	IV	stat (8:00 AM)
3/20	Digoxin 0.25 mg	IV	stat (2:00 PM)
3/20	Digoxin 0.25 mg	IV	stat (8:00 PM)
3/20	Furosemide 40 mg	IV	stat (8:00 AM)
3/21	Furosemide 40 mg	PO	40 mg qd
3/21	Digoxin 0.25 mg	PO	0.25 mg qd

DIETARY ORDERS

Low sodium diet

Figure 6–14

154. The purpose of the furosemide therapy in this patient is to
  A. reduce excess potassium
  B. increase plasma volume
  C. reduce urinary sodium excretion
  D. increase potassium and calcium serum levels
  E. reduce excess sodium and fluid

155. A reasonable daily sodium intake for Mr. Whitfield would be
  A. 2.0 g
  B. 0.2 g
  C. 5.0 g
  D. 12.0 g
  E. 400.0 mg

156. Lab values that should be monitored in a patient on digoxin therapy include
  I. serum creatinine
  II. serum magnesium
  III. serum potassium

  A. I only
  B. III only
  C. I and II only
  D. II and III only
  E. I, II, and III

157. A second serum digoxin level drawn on March 27 is reported as 3.1 ng/mL. What are the possible reason(s) for the increase in the level?
  I. The patient has reached steady-state
  II. The blood was drawn 2 h postdose
  III. The patient's renal function has deteriorated

  A. I only
  B. III only
  C. I and II only
  D. II and III only
  E. I, II, and III

158. On March 21, the physician decides to add captopril to this patient's regimen. A reasonable sig would be

A. 500 mg bid
B. 12.5 mg tid
C. 25 mg qd
D. 50 mg qid
E. 10 mg bid

159. The purpose of using an ACE inhibitor in this patient is to
  I. treat hypertension
  II. achieve afterload reduction
  III. decrease long-term mortality

A. I only
B. III only
C. I and II only
D. II and III only
E. I, II, and III

160. The pharmacist has been asked to educate the patient about the signs and symptoms of digoxin toxicity that require immediate notification of the physician. The pharmacist includes
  I. ringing in the ears
  II. changes in vision
  III. palpitations

A. I only
B. III only
C. I and II only
D. II and III only
E. I, II, and III

161. Which of the following is **NOT** useful in the treatment of acute digoxin toxicity?
  I. Calcium administration
  II. Lidocaine administration
  III. Fab fragment antibodies

A. I only
B. III only
C. I and II only
D. II and III only
E. I, II, and III

162. Which of the following medications interacts with digoxin, resulting in increased digoxin serum concentrations?
- **I.** Amiodarone
- **II.** Verapamil
- **III.** Magnesium hydroxide

- **A.** I only
- **B.** III only
- **C.** I and II only
- **D.** II and III only
- **E.** I, II, and III

163. On March 28, Mr. Whitfield developed a nonproductive, dry cough. Which of the following medications is most likely responsible for this problem?
- **A.** Captopril
- **B.** Furosemide
- **C.** Digoxin
- **D.** A and B
- **E.** All of the above

164. Captopril is discontinued and Mr. Whitfield's cough resolves within 4 days. Which of the following medications would be the most appropriate substitution for captopril?
- **A.** Losartan
- **B.** Verapamil
- **C.** Diltiazem
- **D.** Disopyramide
- **E.** Clonidine

165. What is an appropriate initial dosing regimen for losartan in this patient?
- **A.** 10 mg qd
- **B.** 25 mg qd
- **C.** 100 mg qd
- **D.** 125 mg qd
- **E.** 150 mg qd

166. On discharge, how should Mr. Whitfield be instructed to take his losartan?
- **A.** Only before meals
- **B.** Without regard to meals
- **C.** After meals
- **D.** With food
- **E.** With apple juice

167. What does "stat" mean?
- **A.** At once
- **B.** At 8:00 AM
- **C.** Within the hour
- **D.** Before noon
- **E.** None of the above

DIRECTIONS (Questions 168–178): Refer to the patient profile for Leah Colella (Figure 6–15).

---

168. Which of the following drugs is known **NOT** to interact with warfarin?
- **A.** Acetylsalicylic acid
- **B.** Trimethoprim–sulfamethoxazole
- **C.** Rifampin
- **D.** Diphenhydramine
- **E.** Metronidazole

169. Warfarin is an anticoagulant. Its proposed mechanism of action is that it
- **A.** inhibits platelet synthesis
- **B.** blocks prostaglandin synthesis
- **C.** prohibits absorption of vitamin K
- **D.** binds to fibrinogen
- **E.** inhibits synthesis of vitamin K–dependent clotting factors

MEDICATION PROFILE—INSTITUTION

Name:	Leah Colella
Address:	4624 Hartford Avenue
Age:	65 yr
Weight:	187 lb
Height:	5'8"
Gender:	Female
Allergies:	None
Diagnosis:	Deep vein thrombosis

MEDICATION ORDERS

Date	Drug & Strength	Route	Sig
4/16	Heparin 10,000 units	IV bolus	stat
	Heparin 20,000 units	IV drip	1000 units/hr
4/20	Warfarin 10 mg	PO	one dose (11 AM)
4/21	Warfarin 7.5 mg	PO	one dose (noon)
4/22	Warfarin 5 mg	PO	qd
4/25	DC heparin drip		

Figure 6–15

170. Heparin is another anticoagulant. It is preferred over warfarin on initial diagnosis of which of the following conditions?
     I. Deep-vein thrombosis (DVT)
     II. Pulmonary embolism (PE)
     III. Pregnancy in a patient with a prosthetic heart valve

     A. I only
     B. III only
     C. I and II only
     D. II and III only
     E. I, II, and III

171. After initiating an IV infusion of heparin, the maximum therapeutic response, as measured by the activated partial thromboplastin time (APTT), will be evident in

A. 5 min
B. 5 h
C. 5 days
D. 2 weeks
E. 1 month

172. How many milliliters of heparin (concentration 5,000 units/mL) should be used to prepare a 20,000 units/500 mL 5% dextrose in water?
A. 2 mL
B. 3 mL
C. 4 mL
D. 5 mL
E. 6 mL

173. The heparin admixture as prepared by the pharmacy in Question 172 is delivered to the nursing unit. The nurse wants to know what rate (mL/h) would deliver 1,000 units/h?
A. 20 mL/h
B. 25 mL/h
C. 30 mL/h
D. 35 mL/h
E. 40 mL/h

174. For the treatment of DVT, what is the desired prothrombin time (PT) ratio for warfarin efficacy?
A. 0.5–1.0 times control
B. 0.75–1.5 times control
C. 1.5–2.5 times control
D. 3.0 times control
E. None of the above

175. INR is a standardized method of measuring anticoagulation activity by using the relationship between the INR and the observed PT ratio of rabbit brain thromboplastins. INR stands for
A. international normal-fibrin relationship
B. international normalized ratio
C. internal normal ratio
D. international nomogram relationship
E. none of the above

176. What is the desired INR for the treatment of DVT if ISI is assumed to be 2.5 and PT ratio is 1.3:1.6 using rabbit brain thromboplastin?
   A. 1.0:1.5
   B. 1.5:1.75
   C. 2.0:2.5
   D. 2.0:3.0
   E. 3.0:4.5

177. When counseling Ms. Colella about warfarin therapy, which of the following points should the pharmacist discuss?
   I. Importance of compliance with warfarin therapy
   II. Signs and symptoms of bleeding
   III. Potential drug interactions

   A. I only
   B. III only
   C. I and II only
   D. II and III only
   E. I, II, and III

178. Once Ms. Colella's warfarin therapy is stabilized as an outpatient, what is the recommended interval for laboratory monitoring (INR)?
   A. Daily
   B. Weekly
   C. Monthly
   D. Biannually
   E. Annually

DIRECTIONS (Questions 179–185): Refer to the patient profile for Christopher Scott (Figure 6–16).

---

179. What organism is most commonly isolated from the sputum of cystic fibrosis patients?
   A. *Moraxella catarrhalis*
   B. *Streptococcus pneumoniae*
   C. *Klebsiella penumoniae*
   D. *Pseudomonas aeruginosa*
   E. *Proteus mirabilis*

MEDICATION PROFILE—INSTITUTION

Name:	Christopher Scott
Address:	7928 Mullen
Age:	21 yr
Weight:	102 lb
Gender:	Male
Allergies:	None
Patient Compliant:	SOB, cough, increase in sputum
Admit Diagnosis:	Fever, acute pulmonary infection
Past Med History:	Cystic fibrosis

LABORATORY DIAGNOSTIC TESTS

Hemoglobin	11.2 g/dL
Hematocrit	37.5%
WBC	15,700 cells/mm^3
Serum Creatinine	0.8 mg/dL
Blood glucose	135 mg/dL
PT	14 seconds

ADMISSION ORDERS

Ultrase MT 20	PO	2 caps with meals, 1 cap with snacks
Ranitidine	PO	150 mg bid
Vitamin ADEK	PO	1 tab qd
Dornase alfa	INH	2.5 mg qd
Tobramycin	INH	300 mg q 12 hr
Tobramycin	IV	120 mg q 8 hr
Ticarcillin/clavulanate	IV	3.1 gm q 4 hr
Albuterol	INH	2 inhalations every 4 to 6 hr prn

Figure 6–16

180. Which of the following tests is commonly used to diagnose cystic fibrosis?
   A. Sweat test
   B. Schlicter test
   C. Schilling test
   D. Stress test
   E. Stuart test

181. Pancreatic enzymes are available from many pharmaceutical manufacturers. If this patient was hospitalized in an institution that did not have Ultrase MT 20 on the formulary, a similar product would need to be substituted. That product should have an equivalent amount of which of the following enzymes?
   A. Lipase
   B. Protease
   C. Amylase
   D. Kinase
   E. Collagenase

182. Why is this patient most likely on ranitidine?
   A. Erosive esophagitis
   B. Duodenal ulcer
   C. Systemic mastocytosis
   D. To decrease his pancrease requirement
   E. Gastroesophageal reflux

183. Cystic fibrosis patients commonly have which of the following vitamin deficiencies?
   A. A
   B. D
   C. E
   D. K
   E. All of the above

184. Bleeding and/or bruising indicates a deficiency of which vitamin?
   A. A
   B. D
   C. E
   D. K
   E. All of the above

185. Which of the following information should be provided to a patient using dornase alfa?
   A. Protect the ampules from light
   B. Store the ampules in the refrigerator
   C. Use the entire contents of the ampule or discard remaining solution
   D. Do not mix the product with saline or any other inhalation products
   E. All of the above

186. Which of the following drugs are approved for the treatment of CMV retinitis?
   A. Acyclovir
   B. Valacyclovir
   C. Famciclovir
   D. Ganciclovir
   E. A and B

187. Which laboratory tests are used to diagnose PCP?
   A. Urinalysis
   B. Serum BUN during stress test
   C. CT scan
   D. Sputum/lung biopsy
   E. All of the above

188. What is PCP?
   A. Ameboid larvae found under fingernails that are ingested via mouth
   B. A usually dormant protozoan parasite
   C. Mutant *E coli* found in gingival tissue
   D. Pneumonitis pseudomonas corpuscle, active only if immune function is compromised
   E. A viral infection of the bronchi

DIRECTIONS (Questions 189–262): Each of the questions or incomplete statements below is followed by five suggested answers or completions. Select the **one answer** that is best in each case.

189. Which of the following best describes psoriasis?
  A. Yellow, waxy scales on scalp
  B. Pink, silvery scales on scalp
  C. Yellow, waxy scales on arms and legs
  D. Pink, silvery scales on arms and legs
  E. Pink, silvery scales with underlying inflammation on body

190. Which of the following agents can be safely used during pregnancy?
  A. Atorvastatin
  B. Fluvastatin
  C. Pravastatin
  D. All of the above
  E. None of the above

191. Drugs that may be used for the relief of parkinsonian symptoms include
  I. vecuronium
  II. selegiline
  III. benzotropine mesylate

  A. I only
  B. III only
  C. I and II only
  D. II and III only
  E. I, II, and III

192. Compound W should not be applied to the
  A. face
  B. genitals
  C. toenails
  D. rectum
  E. all of the above

193. Loading doses are recommended when initiating which of the following therapies?
- **A.** Digoxin
- **B.** Amiodarone
- **C.** Sirolimus
- **D.** Esmolol
- **E.** All of the above

194. Patients should be counseled to avoid alcohol while taking which of the following drugs?
- **A.** Metronidazole
- **B.** Disulfiram
- **C.** Griseofulvin
- **C.** Chlorpropamide
- **E.** All of the above

195. Test doses are recommended with which of the following medications?
- **A.** Amphotericin B
- **B.** Lymphocyte immune globulin
- **C.** L-Asparaginase
- **D.** Iron dextran
- **E.** All of the above

196. The body rids itself of ethanol primarily via
- **A.** excretion of unchanged product in the urine
- **B.** hydrolysis in the liver
- **C.** oxidation in the liver
- **D.** reduction in the liver
- **E.** excretion of unchanged product in the lungs

197. Phenobarbital is a known enzyme inducer. This means
- **A.** that phenobarbital is able to inactivate other drugs in a method similar to hepatic enzymes
- **B.** that phenobarbital increases the synthesis of certain enzymes in the liver
- **C.** that adding phenobarbital to a patient's drug regimen will increase plasma drug concentrations
- **D.** all of the above
- **E.** none of the above

198. Acute alcohol ingestion
  A. induces the metabolism of glucose
  B. increases the metabolism of sedative–hypnotic drugs
  C. inhibits the oxidative pathways involved in drug metabolism
  D. does not affect the liver; hepatic changes are observed only after chronic alcoholic ingestion
  E. does none of the above

199. To determine absolute bioavailability of a drug, one must
  A. collect urine for 24–48 h and measure the amount of drug excreted unchanged by the kidney
  B. calculate the area under the serum concentration versus time curve for the IV and extravascular dosage forms
  C. calculate the area under the serum concentration versus time curve for the standard (innovator) oral product and the newly marketed (generic) product
  D. do A and B only
  E. do all of the above

200. Quinidine gluconate and quinidine sulfate may be classified as
  A. chemical equivalents
  B. therapeutic alternatives
  C. chemical and therapeutic equivalents
  D. pharmaceutical equivalents
  E. bioequivalent generic products

201. Which of the following drugs is (are) known to have a substantial first-pass effect after oral administration?
  A. Propranolol
  B. Verapamil
  C. Lidocaine
  D. All of the above
  E. None of the above

202. Urinary alkalinization may be indicated for treatment of an overdosage of
  A. morphine
  B. aminoglycosides
  C. acetaminophen

D. amphetamine
E. phenobarbital

203. Acetylcysteine is used for which of the following conditions?
A. Aspirin overdose
B. Acetaminophen overdose
C. Pulmonary complications of cystic fibrosis
D. B and C
E. A, B, and C

204. Some common patient complaints associated with anticholinergic drugs include all of the following, **EXCEPT**
A. urinary retention
B. shortness of breath
C. blurred vision
D. constipation
E. dry mouth

205. The average half-life of nortriptyline in adults is 35 h. Based on this information, the time to reach steady-state after initiating daily therapy is
A. 70 h
B. 3 days
C. 7–10 days
D. 4–6 weeks
E. indefinite; the patient will never reach steady-state

206. The purpose of fluoride in topical dental products is to
I. prevent tooth staining
II. remove calculus from the tooth surface
III. combine with calcium and phosphorous to strengthen the tooth surface

A. I only
B. III only
C. I and II only
D. II and III only
E. I, II, and III

207. Primatene Mist Inhaler should not be used as self-treatment by patients with which of the following condition(s)?
- **A.** Thyroid disease
- **B.** Heart disease
- **C.** High blood pressure
- **D.** Diabetes
- **E.** All of the above

208. The antiestrogen drug, tamoxifen, is used in the treatment of
- **A.** Hodgkin's disease
- **B.** bladder cancer
- **C.** breast cancer
- **D.** colorectal cancer
- **E.** astrocytoma

209. The most common dose-limiting adverse reaction of anti-neoplastic agents is
- **A.** bone marrow depression
- **B.** cardiac toxicity
- **C.** hepatic toxicity
- **D.** skin necrosis
- **E.** nausea and vomiting

210. Aminobenzoic acid (PABA) is used in which of the following products?
- **A.** Laxatives
- **B.** Cough suppressants
- **C.** Sunscreens
- **D.** Ostomy care
- **E.** All of the above

211. Which of the following statements about quinidine is (are) true?
- **A.** The most common adverse effects are GI reactions
- **B.** It may decrease the effect of digitalis
- **C.** The dosage should be increased in patients with CHF
- **D.** It has a narrow therapeutic index
- **E.** A and D

212. β-Adrenergic blockers
- **A.** block vagal effects on the S–A node
- **B.** decrease conduction through the A–V node

    C. may only be administered orally
    D. are the drugs of choice in patients with sinus bradycardia
    E. are contraindicated in patients receiving digoxin

213. The class of drugs used as first-line agents in panic disorders is
    A. benzodiazepines
    B. MAO inhibitors
    C. tricyclic antidepressants
    D. selective serotonin reuptake inhibitors (SSRIs)
    E. adrenergic blocking agents

214. Which of the following may cause angina?
    A. Atherosclerosis
    B. Anemia
    C. Hyperthyroidism
    D. Hypotension
    E. All of the above

215. The most common side effect of nitrate therapy in the treatment of angina is
    A. chest pain
    B. upset stomach
    C. muscle cramps
    D. headache
    E. all of the above

216. How does carbidopa differ from levodopa?
    A. Carbidopa crosses the blood–brain barrier
    B. Carbidopa is 10 times more effective in controlling symptoms of Parkinson's disease
    C. Carbidopa is safe for use in pregnancy
    D. Carbidopa is available for parenteral administration
    E. Carbidopa alone, when administered, has no effect on symptoms of Parkinson's disease

217. Which of the following antacids is most commonly associated with milk-alkali syndrome?
    A. Aluminum hydroxide
    B. Sodium bicarbonate
    C. Magnesium carbonate
    D. Aluminum phosphate
    E. Magnesium oxide

218. A patient comes into your pharmacy and complains that his urine has become bright orange-red. Which of his current prescription medications may be responsible?
   A. Isoniazid
   B. Ethambutol
   C. Rifampin
   D. Quinidine gluconate
   E. Chloral hydrate

219. The purpose of prescribing a fixed combination of clavulanic acid and amoxicillin is
   A. clavulanic acid enhances the absorption of amoxicillin
   B. clavulanic acid diminishes the gastric side effects of amoxicillin
   C. clavulanic acid provides activity against gram-negative organisms
   D. clavulanic acid is a β-lactamase inhibitor that expands the spectrum of activity of amoxicillin
   E. clavulanic acid inhibits the renal secretion of amoxicillin, thus providing a longer duration of activity

220. Which of the following inhalations should be refrigerated?
   A. Cromolyn sodium
   B. Acetylcysteine
   C. Dornase-alfa
   D. Ipratropium bromide
   E. All of the above

221. Which of the following may increase the absorption of iron?
   I. Ascorbic acid
   II. $AlOH_3$
   III. High-protein meal

   A. I only
   B. III only
   C. I and II only
   D. II and III only
   E. I, II, and III

222. Which of the following iron preparations is **NOT** available in an oral dosage form?

A. Iron dextran
B. Ferrous fumarate
C. Ferrous gluconate
D. Ferrous sulfate
E. Polysaccharide–iron complex

223. What is the recommended daily allowance (RDA) of elemental iron for an adult?
A. 0.1 mg
B. 1.0 mg
C. 10.0 mg
D. 100.0 mg
E. 1.0 g

224. In which of the following conditions is iron supplementation indicated?
I. Primary hemochromatosis
II. Patient receiving multiple blood transfusions
III. Pregnancy

A. I only
B. III only
C. I and II only
D. II and III only
E. I, II, and III

225. Some symptoms of iron deficiency include all of the following **EXCEPT**
A. fatigue
B. constant thirst
C. dystrophy of nails
D. dysphagia
E. dyspnea on exertion

226. Secondary parkinsonism may be caused by
A. chlorpromazine
B. haloperidol
C. reserpine
D. carbon monoxide poisoning
E. all of the above

227. Which of the following is a symptom of parkinsonism?
   A. Pill-rolling movements of the fingers
   B. Constant smile
   C. Dry mouth
   D. Rapid speech
   E. Hearing loss

228. Drugs used to treat parkinsonism work by
   A. stimulating dopamine receptors
   B. decreasing excess acetylcholine
   C. suppressing dopamine production
   D. increasing acetylcholine
   E. A and B

229. Side effects of anticholinergic therapy include
   A. diarrhea
   B. increased salivation
   C. urinary retention
   D. improved memory
   E. increased gastric secretions

230. Which of the following statements about the use of anti-cholinergic agents in the treatment of parkinsonism is (are) FALSE?
   A. Side effects may be potentiated by drugs having anti-cholinergic activity
   B. Patients on combination therapy of levodopa with anti-cholinergism should be monitored for decreased lev-odopa activity due to a shortened gastric emptying time
   C. Patients should be weaned off therapy to avoid exacer-bation of symptoms
   D. Side effects include ataxia, dry mouth, and blurred vision
   E. A and B

231. Which of the following parameters is most indicative of clot-ting in a patient on heparin?
   A. APTT
   B. Urinalysis (for hematuria)
   C. Hematocrit
   D. Platelet count
   E. Stool guaiac

232. Which of the following statements about carbidopa is TRUE?
- **A.** It inhibits peripheral decarboxylation of dopamine
- **B.** A 1:10 ratio contains 250 mg carbidopa and 25 mg levodopa
- **C.** The incidence of nausea and vomiting may be increased with the combination
- **D.** It reduces the amount of required levodopa by 60–75%
- **E.** None of the above

233. Which of the following is (are) possible side effects of bromocriptine therapy?
- **A.** First-dose phenomenon
- **B.** Hypertension
- **C.** Increased alertness
- **D.** Decreased GI function
- **E.** All of the above

234. Which of the following statements is (are) TRUE about drug holidays for parkinsonism therapy?
- **A.** They may benefit patients who lose effectiveness with long-term therapy
- **B.** They may result in a reduction in the dose required to control the symptoms
- **C.** They may produce more on–off episodes
- **D.** A and B
- **E.** The holiday period should last approximately 1 month

235. Which of the following may be the cause for lack of therapeutic effectiveness of an antibiotic?
- **A.** Misdiagnosis
- **B.** Improper drug regimen
- **C.** Inappropriate choice of antibiotic
- **D.** Microbial resistance
- **E.** All of the above

236. Which of the following are considered shorter acting benzodiazepines?
- **A.** Clonazepam
- **B.** Diazepam
- **C.** Alprazolam
- **D.** A and B
- **E.** A, B, and C

237. Which of the following drugs has been associated with Stevens-Johnson syndrome?
   A. Phenytoin
   B. Allopurinol
   C. Lamotrigine
   D. Sulfamethoxazole–trimethoprim
   E. All of the above

238. Which of the following penicillins has a long duration of action?
   A. Oxacillin
   B. Amoxicillin
   C. Penicillin G procaine
   D. Penicillin G benzathine
   E. C and D

239. Which of the following should a pharmacist discuss with a patient when dispensing a prescription for nitroglycerin patches for the first time?
   I. The possibility that headaches and/or dizziness may accompany the initiation of therapy
   II. The possibility that contact dermatitis may occur
   III. Daily rotation of application sites

   A. I only
   B. III only
   C. I and II only
   D. II and III only
   E. I, II, and III

240. An appropriate dose of nitroglycerin prescribed in a transdermal delivery system would be
   A. 15 mg/24 h
   B. 0.15 mg/24 h
   C. 100 mg/12 h
   D. 0.5 mg/24 h
   E. 0.500 g/24 h

241. The principal pharmacologic action of nitroglycerin involves a
   A. decrease in the heart rate
   B. lengthening of ejection time in the cardiac cycle

C. decrease in inotropic effect
D. relaxation of vascular smooth muscle
E. reduction in total blood volume

242. Which of the following agents would **NOT** be indicated for a patient with angina?
A. Isosorbide
B. Flecainide
C. Nifedipine
D. Inderal
E. Diltiazem

243. All of the following may be symptoms of a myocardial infarction **EXCEPT**
A. myalgia, mydriasis, and nocturia
B. agitated behavior and ashen pallor
C. nausea, sweating, and dyspnea
D. heartburn, fainting, and skipped beats
E. dental and neck pain, no relief from nitroglycerin

244. Which needle has the largest diameter?
A. 16 gauge
B. 18 gauge
C. 21 gauge
D. 25 gauge
E. 27 gauge

245. Which of the following may be factors in digoxin toxicity?
A. Hypokalemia
B. Drug interactions
C. Hypothyroidism
D. Renal insufficiency
E. All of the above

246. Which of the following antiarrhythmic drugs are associated with cinchonism?
A. Lidocaine
B. Mexiletine
C. Tocainide
D. Quinidine
E. Moricizine

247. Which of the following labs should be drawn whenever a digoxin level is drawn?

A. Calcium
B. Potassium
C. Sodium
D. Chloride
E. Phosphate

248. Which of the following conditions may predispose a patient to contract pulmonary tuberculosis?

A. HIV infection
B. Silicosis
C. Imprisonment
D. Crowded living conditions
E. All of the above

249. Which of the following statements generally applies to cancer chemotherapy?

   I. The use of a single antineoplastic drug is preferable in the treatment of leukemias and lymphomas to minimize side effects

  II. The fraction of tumor cells killed is related to drug dose and may be described by a first-order process

 III. Drug therapy should be initiated when the tumor growth fraction is high

A. I only
B. III only
C. I and II only
D. II and III only
E. I, II, and III

250. Which of the following agents has the greatest potential to cause bone marrow suppression?

A. Nitrogen mustard
B. Vincristine
C. Fluoxymesterone
D. Levamisole
E. Tamoxifen

251. The administration of indomethacin and aspirin are con-
traindicated in patients receiving high-dose methotrexate
therapy because they
  I. inhibit renal elimination of unchanged methotrexate
 II. decrease the half-life of methotrexate
III. interfere with the mechanism of action of methotrexate

  A. I only
  B. III only
  C. I and II only
  D. II and III only
  E. I, II, and III

252. An appropriate dose of methotrexate for the treatment of
rheumatoid arthritis is
  A. 0.5 mg qd
  B. 1.0 g once weekly
  C. 7.5 mg once weekly
  D. 7.5 mg qid
  E. 250.0 mg qod

253. Therapeutic response to methotrexate in patients with rheu-
matoid arthritis is usually observed within
  A. 1 h, if administered IV
  B. 3–6 hours
  C. 3–6 days
  D. 3–6 weeks
  E. 3–6 months

254. All of the following statements pertain to methotrexate
EXCEPT
  A. methotrexate does not pass from the blood into the cere-
brospinal fluid
  B. oral and GI mucosal ulceration occur frequently
  C. the mechanism of action of methotrexate in cancer
chemotherapy involves inhibition of tetrahydrofolate
reduction
  D. hepatotoxicity is more frequent with daily long-term
therapy than with intermittent therapy
  E. methotrexate is rapidly and completely absorbed after
oral administration

255. Sixty mg methotrexate was inadvertently administered IV to the wrong patient. The appropriate antidote would be
- **A.** 5 mg folic acid, IV
- **B.** 60 mg folvite, IV
- **C.** 60 mg folic acid, IV
- **D.** 60 mg leucovorin calcium, IV
- **E.** 300 mg leucovorin calcium, IV

256. Cyclophosphamide is categorized as a (an)
- **A.** purine antagonist
- **B.** alkylating agent
- **C.** cytotoxic glycopeptide antibiotic
- **D.** synthetic pyrimidine nucleoside
- **E.** a rimidine antagonist

257. All of the following are known side effects of doxorubicin therapy **EXCEPT**
- **A.** stomatitis and esophagitis
- **B.** hemorrhagic cystitis
- **C.** leukopenia
- **D.** alopecia
- **E.** congestive heart failure

258. OTC products used to treat seborrhea are similar to those used in the treatment of psoriasis **EXCEPT**
- **A.** the antiseborrhetics are used in higher concentration
- **B.** the antiseborrhetics are generally used as shampoos
- **C.** the antiseborrhetics require a prescription
- **D.** the antiseborrhetics require an occlusive dressing to be effective
- **E.** A and D

259. The goal of treatment for psoriasis is
- **A.** to remove unsightly scales
- **B.** to reduce cell turnover
- **C.** to add moisture to skin
- **D.** A and B
- **E.** A, B, and C

260. Which of the following may promote fungal or yeast infections on the body?
- **A.** Immunosuppression
- **B.** Moisture

C. Warmth
D. Broad-spectrum antibiotics
E. All of the above

261. A pyoderma may be defined as
A. a hemorrhoid
B. a fungal infection of the nail
C. a bacterial infection of the skin
D. a cold sore
E. none of the above

262. Ringworm may be best described as
A. a worm infestation of the skin
B. a bacterial infection
C. a tinea infection
D. scabies
E. B and C

Authors' Note: Although this text has been updated in all sections with new products, this next section briefly summarizes new drugs, dosage forms, or approved indications that have been marketed in the United States during 1998 through October 2001.

DIRECTIONS (Questions 263–270) *Oncology Medications:* From the following list, select the most appropriate therapy for the condition named.

A. Gemtuzumab
B. Capectabine
C. Valrubicin
D. Temozolomide
E. Triptorelin

263. Prostate cancer

264. Acute myeloid leukemia

265. Metastatic breast cancer

266. BCG carcinoma

267. Astrocytoma

DIRECTIONS (Questions 268–270): From the following list, select the most appropriate therapy for the condition named.

    A. Toremifene
    B. Imatinib
    C. Alitretinoin

268. Chronic myelogenous leukemia

269. Kaposi sarcoma cutaneous lesions

270. Advanced breast cancer

DIRECTIONS (Questions 270-275) *Psychiatric/Neurology Medications:* From the following list, select the most appropriate therapy for the condition named.

    A. Citalopram
    B. Rivastigamine
    C. Ziprasidone
    D. Oxcarbazepine
    E. Levetiracetam

271. Depression

272. Alzheimer's disease

273. Schizophrenia

274. Partial onset seizures in adults and children

275. Partial seizures in adults

DIRECTIONS (Questions 276–280) *Anti-Infective Medications:* From the following list, select the most appropriate therapy for the condition named.

    A. Amprenavir
    B. Fomivirsen
    C. Dalfopristin/quinupristin
    D. Rifapentine
    E. Cefditoren

276. Acute bacterial infections

277. Vancomycin-resistant enterococcus

278. Tuberculosis

279. CMV retinitis

280. AIDS (protease inhibitor)

DIRECTIONS (Questions 281–285) *Cardiovascular/Hematologic Medications:* From the following list, select the most appropriate therapy for the condition named.

    A. Argatroban
    B. Candesartan
    C. Dofetilide
    D. Nesiritide
    E. Tirofiban

281. Anticoagulant for hemodialysis patients

282. CHF

283. Hypertension (angiotensin II antagonist)

284. Atrial fibrillation

285. Acute coronary syndrome

DIRECTIONS (Questions 286–290) *Miscellaneous Medications:* From the following list, select the most appropriate therapy for the condition named.

    A. Sirolimus
    B. Brinzolamide
    C. Montelukast
    D. Rofecoxib
    E. Formoterol

286. Prophylaxis for organ transplant

287. Asthma

288. COPD

289. Osteoarthritis

290. Open angle glaucoma

DIRECTIONS (Questions 291-295) *Miscellaneous Medications:* From the following list, select the most appropriate therapy for the condition named.

    A. Zaleplon
    B. Nitric oxide
    C. Entacapone
    D. Rizatriptan
    E. Exemestane

291. Pulmonary hypertension

292. Insomnia

293. Parkinson's disease

294. Acute migraine

295. Advanced breast cancer

DIRECTIONS (Questions 296-300) *Miscellaneous Medications:* From the following list, select the most appropriate therapy for the condition named.

   A. Galantamine
   B. Almotriptan
   C. Budenoside
   D. Valganciclovir
   E. Esomperazole

296. Alzheimer's disease

297. CMV retinitis

298. Crohn's disease

299. Acute migraine

300. Erosive esophagitis

Clinical Pharmacy

Answers and Discussion

1. **(D)** Two million units of penicillin G potassium contains approximately 130 mg potassium. Ms. Grant has chronic renal failure with an elevated serum potassium (normal range is 3.5 to 5 mEq/L). The Jarisch–Herxheimer reaction (chills, fever, headache, joint pain) occurs in patients with secondary syphilis after the first injection of penicillin.

2. **(D)** The respiratory symptoms described as part of this patient's allergic reaction to penicillin suggest a serious, possibly life-threatening allergy. Aminopenicillins, such as ampicillin, and cefazolin (a first-generation cephalosporin) would not be recommended in this patient because of potential cross allergenicity.

3. **(B)** Normal adult serum creatinine levels range from 0.7 to 1.5 mg/dL. Milligrams per deciliter (mg/dL) and milligrams percent (mg%) are equivalent units.

4. **(D)** Normal creatinine clearance values range from 100 to 125 mL/min.

5. **(C)** For most renally excreted drugs, it is not necessary to adjust dosage until the estimated creatinine clearance falls below 50 mL/min.

6. **(D)** For a patient with normal renal function, the usual dose of gentamicin is 1.5 mg/kg q 8 h. This patient has a creatinine clearance that is less than one-quarter normal. The dosing interval must be extended in order to prevent nephrotoxicity. Gentamicin is poorly absorbed orally and therefore is not administered by the oral route to treat systemic infections.

7. **(A)** The half-life of gentamicin in adult patients with normal renal function varies from 2–4 hours. In anuric patients, the half-life is greater than 30 hours.

8. **(E)** Gentamicin exhibits first-order elimination. The elimination of gentamicin is prolonged in patients with chronic renal failure.

9. **(E)** Ciprofloxacin, imipenem, and aztreonam are all effective antibiotics against gram-negative organisms. Dosage adjustment is necessary for all three agents in patients with renal impairment.

10. **(B)** Allopurinol is frequently prescribed for patients with chronic renal failure to diminish the uric acid load to the kidney.

11. **(C)** Antacids containing sodium bicarbonate and magnesium are contraindicated in patients with renal failure.

12. **(B)** Oral ciprofloxacin is available as 250, 500, and 750 mg tablets. The IV dose is 400 mg.

13. **(A)** Patients with a known sulfa sensitivity may experience a cross reaction when receiving a thiazide.

14. **(B)** Thiazide diuretics exert their effect at the distal portion of the loop of Henle. Furosemide exerts its effect at the ascending loop of Henle.

15. **(A)** Postmenopausal women not receiving estrogen replacement therapy require a calcium intake of 1–1.5 g/d to maintain positive calcium balance and prevent osteoporosis.

16. (B) Alendronate, a bisphosphonate, inhibits bone resorption through direct and indirect actions on osteoclasts.

17. (C) To facilitate absorption and minimize esophageal irritation, alendronate must be taken on an empty stomach with a full glass of plain water; patients should not lie down for a minimum of 30 min after administration.

18. (E) Divalent trivalent cations chelate with ciprofloxacin in the GI tract and reduce bioavailability of the antibiotic if administered concurrently.

19. (C) Cromolyn is available commercially as an oral inhalant, oral capsule, metered-dose inhalant, and powder inhalant. There is no parenteral dosage form.

20. (D) Cromolyn is a mast-cell stabilizer.

21. (A) Patients with moderate asthma have a PEFR of 60–80% of normal. Patients with mild asthma have a PEFR >80%.

22. (E) All three steps are necessary for efficient drug delivery.

23. (D) Tolerance can develop to the beta agonists, but they are not addicting.

24. (D) Beta agonists relax bronchial smooth muscle and may affect mediator release from mast cells.

25. (B) Salmeterol is a long-acting beta agonist. Because of a delayed onset of action, it should not be used for treatment of acute exacerbations of asthma.

26. (E) Some of the common medications that may trigger asthma are aspirin, nonsteroidal anti-inflammatory agents, and beta blockers.

27. (C) Inhaled short acting beta-2 agonists are most effective for prevention of exercise-induced asthma. Regular use of these agents on a scheduled basis is not recommended. They should be used only for acute bronchospasm or prevention of exercise-induced asthma.

28. **(A)** Patients should be instructed to rinse their mouths after using corticosteroid oral inhalers to reduce the incidence of oral candidiasis.

29. **(C)** The patient weighs 79 lbs (36 kg). The commercial product that would deliver the best approximation of the desired dose is 250 mg/5 mL.

30. **(C)** Concomitant use of clarithromycin and theophylline may result in elevated theophylline serum levels. Theophylline levels should be checked while the patient is receiving clarithromycin and after the antibiotic is discontinued. An alternative antibiotic may be advisable.

31. **(B)** The generic name of Vanceril is beclomethasone.

32. **(E)** Non–insulin-dependent diabetics are at risk for hypertension, hyperlipidemia, nephropathy, and neuropathy.

33. **(D)** Acarbose inhibits the enzyme responsible for the breakdown of starch and sucrose in the small intestines.

34. **(B)** Acarbose exerts its effects in the small intestines. Absorption is not necessary for therapeutic activity.

35. **(B)** Sibutramine is contraindicated in patients with poorly controlled hypertension. Although its use is also contraindicated concurrently with MAO inhibitors, the patient is not currently taking an MAO inhibitor, and has not within the last two weeks.

36. **(B)** Diabetic patients are at increased risk of developing neuropathy. Typical analgesic therapy often is not fully effective in relieving symptoms. Several antidepressants and anticonvulsants are used to treat neuropathic syndromes, including amitriptyline, fluoxetine, carbamazepine, and gabapentin.

37. (C) The duration of action of chlorpropamide can be up to 60 h. This long duration can lead to serious side effects and overdose in patients with renal and hepatic impairment.

38. (E) Low blood sugar produces blurred vision, headache, confusion, weakness, diaphoresis, and irritability.

39. (A) Treatment of hypoglycemia usually involves administration of 10–20 g of rapidly absorbed carbohydrate. If the patient is unconscious, administer parenteral glucagon or glucose.

40. (C) Daily monitoring of the skin, especially on the feet, is necessary in diabetic patients. They should never attempt self-treatment of corns and calluses because of the risk of infection and gangrene.

41. (E) Acetone breath and dry skin are classic symptoms of diabetic ketoacidosis.

42. (D) Extremely high blood glucose levels may be observed in hyperglycemic coma.

43. (E) Diabetic neuropathy involves both the autonomic and peripheral nervous systems.

44. (E) Thiazide diuretics may induce hyperglycemia. Propranolol is a beta blocker that masks the symptoms of hypoglycemia and may contribute to hypoglycemia. By changing the antihypertensive regimen, the patient is at risk for hypoglycemia unless blood sugars are monitored closely.

45. (B) ACE inhibitors such as captopril (Capoten) have no effect on glucose tolerance and are recommended therapy in patients with diabetic nephropathy. Atenolol (Tenormin) and metoprolol (Lopressor) are beta blockers that may potentiate hypoglycemia in diabetic patients.

46. (B) Ortho-Novum 777 is a triphasic oral contraceptive— the estrogen (ethinyl estradiol) amount remains the same and the progestin (norethindrone) amount varies throughout the cycle. A biphasic oral contraceptive contains the same amount of estrogen for the first part of the cycle (21 days). A decreased progestin/estrogen ratio in the first half of the cycle allows endometrial proliferation. An increased ratio in the second half provides adequate secretory development. A monophasic oral contraceptive maintains a fixed ratio of estrogen/progestin throughout the cycle.

47. (E) All three items should be discussed with the patient. In addition, the patient should be instructed on what to do if a dose is missed and to contact their physician if chronic breakthrough bleeding occurs.

48. (A) The patient should be instructed to take 2 tablets that day and to continue with the cycle.

49. (E) Patients taking tetracycline should avoid chronic sunlight exposure because photosensitivity is associated with therapy. The simultaneous ingestion of dairy products high in calcium interferes with tetracycline absorption via chelation and should be avoided. Coadministration of tetracycline with oral contraceptives (OCs) may decrease their pharmacologic effects, possibly due to altered steroid gut metabolism as a result of changes in intestinal flora. Alternative or additional methods of contraception are advisable.

50. (C) Vaginal tablets are meant to be administered via the applicator provided with the prescription. They are not to be crushed before insertion into the applicator.

51. (B) Chronic antibiotic regimens such as tetracycline may predispose patients to yeast infections. The amoxicillin regimen was not causally related because it was an acute regimen approximately 9 months prior to the event. OCs are not associated with an increased risk of yeast infections.

52. (A) Prenatal vitamins have been prescribed for the patient. Oral contraceptives have an FDA pregnancy rating of X. Their use may lead to increased fetal risk and is contraindicated during pregnancy.

53. (E) The patient is allergic to aspirin. Ascriptin, Bayer Plus, and Excedrin all contain aspirin.

54. (B) Most urinary tract infections (UTIs) are caused by *Escherichia coli.* Penicillin or cephalosporins are considered to be safe during pregnancy and *E coli* usually is sensitive to one of these agents. Tetracycline, trimethoprim, and ciprofloxacin are contraindicated during pregnancy. Vancomycin is not absorbed orally and is thus inappropriate for a UTI.

55. (B) Stomach upset is a common event during pregnancy. Limited use of antacids may be recommended.

56. (E) None of the drugs mentioned should be recommended; most antihistamines are excreted in significant amounts into breast milk. Thus, antihistamine therapy is contraindicated in nursing mothers.

57. (C) Oral contraception may be started as early as 4–6 weeks at the first postpartum examination in nonnursing mothers, regardless of whether spontaneous menstruation has occurred.

58. (A) Although ibuprofen is used for all these indications, this dosage represents the maximum daily recommendation (3.2 g/d) and is most commonly used in the treatment of rheumatoid arthritis. A typical regimen for the treatment of dysmenorrhea is 400 mg q 4 h PRN. Fever typically responds to OTC dosage regimens: 200 mg q 4–6 h while symptoms persist.

59. (C) GI complaints are the most common side effects associated with ibuprofen use. This patient may be at particular risk because of the high dosage. The bioavailability of ibuprofen is not significantly affected by the concurrent administration of food or antacids.

60. (D) The primary mechanism of action of ibuprofen is inhibition of prostaglandin synthesis by blocking the cyclooxygenase pathway. Prostaglandins have many complex effects

on the body, including the stimulation of platelet aggregation, maintenance of blood flow to the kidneys, promotion of
inflammatory response, and protection of the GI mucosa.

61. (E) Because Ms. Whitfield is on a high NSAID regimen,
she is at risk for the development of a peptic ulcer or other
serious GI toxicity. The use of an OTC product would only
delay appropriate medical attention. Referral to her physician would be the recommended action in this case.

62. (C) Misoprostol should be taken with food to lessen stomach distress and decrease the incidence of diarrhea.

63. (A) Misoprostol is indicated for the prevention of NSAID-
induced gastric ulcers in patients who are at high risk for the
development of this problem.

64. (C) Misoprostol is a synthetic prostaglandin E1 analog that
inhibits gastric acid secretion, has mucosal protective properties, and increases GI bicarbonate and mucus production.

65. (A) Although all of these symptoms are side effects of
misoprostol therapy, diarrhea is the most common event
associated with this agent and occurs in approximately
13–40% of patients. This effect usually occurs early and
resolves with continued therapy. Diarrhea requires discontinuation in approximately 2% of patients. Other side effects
such as dysmenorrhea, headache, cramps, and constipation
occur in less than 3% of patients.

66. (E) Misoprostol has an FDA pregnancy category rating of
X and should not be taken during pregnancy. This drug may
also cause miscarriage because of its ability to induce uterine contractions. Thus, the patient should have a negative
serum pregnancy test within 2 weeks prior to beginning therapy with misoprostol and only begin therapy on the second
or third day of the next normal menstrual period.

67. (E) Misoprostol therapy should be continued for the life of
the NSAID therapy, but should be discontinued if the patient
becomes pregnant.

68. (C) Sucralfate and antacids interfere with the GI absorption of ciprofloxacin and should be administered 2–4 h before or after ciprofloxacin.

69. (E) Smoking adversely effects the GI mucosa via all the methods mentioned. Smokers are therefore at a higher risk of developing peptic ulcer disease, which is slower to heal and has a higher incidence of recurrence. Smoking should be discouraged in this patient.

70. (E) Typical duodenal pain is described as a gnawing or burning sensation near the xyphoid. Patients often awaken late at night with pain that disappears by morning. Food often relieves the pain.

71. (C) Antacids neutralize existing gastric acid secreted by the parietal cells and increase the pH of the stomach and duodenal bulb. Antacids also inhibit the conversion of pepsinogen to pepsin by increasing pH. Antacids do not inhibit gastric acid secretion.

72. (B) Histamine-2 receptor antagonists inhibit gastric acid secretion by competitively blocking histamine-2 receptors on the parietal cell. Suppression of nocturnal and basal gastric acid secretion approximates 90%.

73. (D) Sucralfate does not reduce or neutralize gastric acid. Once in the stomach it dissolves, releasing aluminum, which forms a viscous gel that has a strong negative charge and binds to positively charged chemical groups, including defective mucosa. Sucralfate primarily acts as a cytoprotectant.

74. (E) All these foods promote gastric secretion and affect sphincter tone.

75. (C) Blood in vomitus (red or coffee ground) and blood in stools (black, tarry stools) are indicative of active upper GI bleeding. Patients with these symptoms should be referred to physician for immediate attention. Epistaxis (nosebleeds) are not correlated with GI bleeding.

76. (C) Because clarithromycin has been prescribed at the same time as H2 antagonist therapy it is most likely for *H pylori*. Duodenal ulcers have been related to infection with *H pylori,* a spiral-shaped bacterium that colonizes the epithelial cells of the stomach mucosal lining. Eradication with dual or triple therapy including histamine-2 antagonists, bismuth subcitrate, and clarithromycin have been effective in promoting healing and preventing recurrence.

77. (D) Clarithromycin is a macrolide antibiotic that reversibly binds to the P site of the 50S ribosomal subunit of susceptible organisms and inhibits RNA-dependent protein synthesis. Other drugs in this class include erythromycin, azithromycin, and troleandomycin.

78. (B) The fexofenadine prescription is written for too high a dose. Typical dosage for fexofenadine to treat allergic rhinitis or urticaria is 60 mg bid or 180 mg once daily.

79. (C) Celecoxib is contraindicated for use in patients with a allergic history to celecoxib, sulfonamides, aspirin or other NSAIDs. The product labeling also warns against use in patients with a history of GI disease. Thus, this drug is not an appropriate choice for this patient.

80. (D) Celecoxib is approved for treatment of pain associated with osteoarthritis and rheumatoid arthritis. It is also used to reduce the number of adenomatous colorectal polyps in patients with familial adenomatous polypsis as adjunct therapy to usual care. It is not FDA approved for acute pain syndromes.

81. (B) Although rofecoxib can be used in patients with sulfonamide allergies, it along with aspirin and indomethacin should not be used in patients with active ulcer disease. Based on this data, acetaminophen would be a likely initial choice. However, the patient may need to be reevaluated if acetaminophen does not provide enough analgesia coverage.

82. (B) Citalopram as the brand product Celexa is indicated for the treatment of depression.

83. (B) PMDD is the abbreviation for premenstrual dysphoric disorder.

84. (B) Fluoxetine as the brand product Sarafem is indicated for treatment of PMDD.

85. (A) Initially, the starting dose for fluoxetine (Sarafem) in patients with PMDD is 20 mg/d. Doses of 60 mg/d are also effective; however, no significant added benefit compared to 20 mg/d is obtained. Efficacy is maintained for up to 6 months with a dose of 20 mg/d. Reevaluate patients periodically to determine the need for continued treatment. The maximum dose should not exceed 80 mg/d.

86. (B) Fluoxetine is a cytochrome P450IID6 (CYP2D6) inhibitor and thus inhibits dextromethorphan metabolism. Serotonin syndrome, characterized by restlessness, myoclonus, and changes in mental status, is a possibility with the combined use of dextromethorphan and serotonergic agents. Serotonin syndrome has been reported when dextromethorphan has been taken concurrently with fluoxetine or other serotonin specific reuptake inhibitors.

87. (A) Because sibutramine and its some of its metabolites inhibit the reuptake of norepinephrine, dopamine, and serotonin, serotonin syndrome may result if sibutramine is given concurrently with a selective serotonin reuptake inhibitor. Coadministration of sibutramine and selective serotonin reuptake inhibitors is not recommended via the package insert labeling of sibutramine.

88. (E) Phenytoin chewable tablets contain phenytoin acid, which is 100% phenytoin.

89. (D) Phenytoin follows nonlinear saturable kinetics. The apparent half-life of the drug changes with the dose. If the daily dose is below the maximum capacity of the enzymes responsible for metabolizing phenytoin, steady state levels should be 90% of maximum within 30 days. Weekly blood level determinations are recommended during the first month of therapy.

90. (E) Common dose-related adverse reactions to phenytoin include nystagmus, ataxia, confusion, drowsiness, gingival hyperplasia, and choreiform movements.

91. (C) Dilantin Kapseals is the only product currently approved for once daily dosing because of its extended absorption characteristics.

92. (D) Carbamazepine causes nausea and vomiting in a significant number of patients, particularly at high doses. Food does not appear to affect the total amount of drug absorbed. Anticonvulsants in general cause drowsiness.

93. (B) Monthly monitoring of complete blood counts is recommended for patients receiving carbamazepine. Carbamazepine has been reported to cause aplastic anemia, transient leukopenia, and agranulocytosis.

94. (C) Status epilepticus is generally defined as repeated generalized seizures with no recovery of the postictal state between seizures.

95. (D) In status epilepticus, it is critical to maintain an unobstructed airway, initiate a dextrose infusion if the cause is unknown, and administer diazepam 10 mg IV.

96. (A) Fosphenytoin is a prodrug of phenytoin and intended for parenteral administration (IM or IV). The conversion half-life of fosphenytoin to phenytoin is approximately 15 min. After IM administration, peak concentrations occur at approximately 30 min postdose.

97. (A) For each millimole of fosphenytoin administered, 1 mmol of phenytoin is produced. Fosphenytoin is monitored via total plasma phenytoin concentrations.

98. (C) Steady state levels of anticonvulsants are necessary to ensure safe and effective therapy. Therapeutic phenytoin concentrations range from 10–20 µg/mL.

99. (C)   The amounts and concentrations of fosphenytoin are expressed in terms of phenytoin sodium equivalents (PE) and may reduce the incidence of medication errors or confusion between this product and phenytoin.

100. (B)   Carbamazepine is a well-known hepatic enzyme inducer of drug metabolism. It also induces its own metabolism (autoinducer) and is known to induce the metabolism of phenytoin, often requiring dosage adjustments within 2–4 weeks of being added or discontinued.

101. (E)   Phenytoin has several significant drug interactions that, when given concurrently, may cause phenytoin toxicity.

102. (E)   Erythromycin is also a hepatic enzyme inhibitor and has been reported to increase carbamazepine serum concentrations.

103. (A)   Barbiturates suppress transmission across the synapses and thereby raise the seizure threshold.

104. (B)   Daily doses of phenobarbital produce serum levels of 15–35 µg/mL. This is generally adequate to control seizures.

105. (B)   Enzyme induction increases the amount of enzyme in the liver, thereby increasing the rate of drug metabolism.

106. (D)   Carbohydrates provide the primary source of energy. The most common form of carbohydrate used in parenteral nutrition is dextrose.

107. (B)   There are 100 grams in 1 L of 10% dextrose.

108. (D)   Lipid emulsion is commercially available in 10%, 20%, and 30% concentrations. However, the 30% emulsion is only intended to be used in the preparation of parenteral nutrition, not for direct administration to the patient.

109. (B)   Twenty percent dextrose is hypertonic and will cause damage to the vein if administered peripherally.

110. (C) To decrease the chance of precipitation, published guidelines limiting the amounts of phosphorus and calcium should be carefully followed. In addition, when mixing the solution, one of these minerals should be added last so that the product is as dilute as possible and the risk of precipitation is minimized.

111. (E) All influence calcium and phosphate incompatibility.

112. (E) All are true.

113. (B) Infliximab, a chimeric monoclonal antibody to tumor necrosis factor-alpha (TNF-α), is approved for use in patients with moderate-to-severe disease/draining enterocutaneous fistulae refractory to conventional treatment (e.g., prednisone, azathioprine, mercaptopurine, and aminosalicylates).

114. (A) Infliximab is also used in rheumatoid arthritis.

115. (D) The recommended infliximab dose is 5 mg/kg IV infusion over 2 h. Normal saline is used as infusion diluent.

116. (E) Serious infections, including disseminated tuberculosis and sepsis have been associated with infliximab therapy. In October 2001 the FDA notified health professionals that tuberculosis and other serious opportunistic infections, including histoplasmosis, listeriosis, and pneumocystosis, have been reported in both clinical research and postmarking surveillance. Some of these infections have been fatal. The manufacturer has added a boxed warning to the labeling of the product regarding this concern.

117. (A) Because of a decreased immune response in patients receiving infliximab, live vaccines are not recommended.

118. (C) Many signs and symptoms of otitis media and meningitis overlap. A stiff neck is not a typical presentation for otitis media and would signify the need to examine the child to rule out meningitis. Twenty-five percent of children with *Haemophilus influenzae* otitis media also have signs and symptoms of bacteremia or meningitis.

119. (B) Clavulanic acid is a beta-lactamase inhibitor that will improve coverage against beta-lactamase producing bacteria usually resistant to ampicillin–amoxicillin.

120. (D) Ciprofloxacin is *not* recommended for use in children or pregnant patients because of potential adverse effects in developing limbs.

121. (C) The suspension must be refrigerated and discarded after 10 days. Food intake does not effect amoxicillin–clavulanate absorption. Diarrhea and loose stools are common side effects of amoxicillin–clavulanate therapy.

122. (E) All three explanations are common reasons for the need for retreatment of otitis media. Recurrent infections are not unusual in pediatric patients.

123. (D) Hashimoto's thyroiditis is an inflammation of the thyroid gland and the most common cause of hypothyroidism.

124. (E) Liotrix is a 4:1 combination of T_4:T_3 designed to mimic natural hormone ratios in the body.

125. (E) If the replacement dose is adequate, maximal effects from replacement therapy should be seen in 4–8 weeks.

126. (B) The USP requirement for desiccated thyroid states that it must contain between 0.17% and 0.23% organic iodine. The ratio of T_3 to T_4 can vary.

127. (C) Eighty percent of total T_3 production is the result of conversion of T_4 to T_3 in the periphery. Many drugs interact with levothyroxine. For example, cholestyramine, iron products, and antacids bind levothyroxine in the GI tract and decrease bioavailability if given concurrently.

128. (E) Abrupt onset and acute symptoms of thirst, urination, and fatigue are indicative of type I diabetes.

129. (E) Any of these findings is indicative of diabetes.

130. **(A)** Complex carbohydrates provide a uniform release of glucose into the blood, thus preventing wide swings in insulin levels.

131. **(D)** Human insulin is derived from recombinant DNA technology.

132. **(E)** Lente insulin is an intermediate acting insulin with an onset of 1.5–3 h.

133. **(A)** Initial doses of insulin are routinely based on total body weight.

134. **(A)** Patients using <50 units insulin per dose should use the 1/2 cc syringe.

135. **(E)** In addition to these instructions, patients should be reminded to check expiration dates on insulin vials before use.

136. **(E)** Any stress condition on the body that is not taken into account in the daily insulin dose can cause ketoacidosis.

137. **(E)** Diabetic coma from elevated blood glucose levels produces all of these symptoms.

138. **(E)** Fluid and electrolyte replacement and regular insulin will reverse diabetic coma.

139. **(C)** Hypertension is common in patients with diabetes.

140. **(A)** Regular insulin, with an onset of action of 30–60 min, should be used to control preprandial hyperglycemia.

141. **(D)** Diazepam is the drug of choice in status epilepticus. Phenytoin should not be administered IV push because of venous irritation and potential cardiac adverse effects.

142. **(D)** Ethanol is a competitive substrate for alcohol dehydrogenase, preventing the metabolism of methanol to its toxic

metabolite, formic acid. The unchanged methanol is then renally excreted.

143. **(B)** This calculation can be solved using alligation or algebra: Let x = the volume of 95% alcohol needed—then

$$95(x) + 5(1000 - x) = 10 (1000)$$

144. **(E)** Although lithium is best known as an antimanic, it also possesses some antidepressant properties.

145. **(C)** The usual therapeutic range of lithium is 0.5–1.5 mEq/L.

146. **(D)** Hand tremors are the most common lithium side effect. Lithium also causes diarrhea and GI distress, which may be dose-related.

147. **(E)** Adverse GI effects can be minimized if taken with meals. Patient must maintain fluid intake because of the propensity of lithium to cause polyuria.

148. **(A)** It usually takes 10–21 days to observe optimal response to a lithium dosage regimen.

149. **(B)** Valproic acid is an effective agent for the control of absence seizures.

150. **(A)** The generic name of Prozac is fluoxetine. Sertraline and paroxetine are also serotonin reuptake inhibitors.

151. **(B)** Fluoxetine inhibits the metabolism of valproic acid. It may also lead to additive CNS side effects.

152. **(C)** Cimetidine inhibits the metabolism of valproic acid and should be avoided if possible.

153. **(C)** Digoxin is a cardiac glycoside with a very long half-life (30–40 h in a patient with normal renal function). It takes about 1 week to reach steady-state levels if a patient is started directly on an oral maintenance dosing regimen. To achieve therapeutic body levels more quickly, a 1-day IV or

2-day oral loading dose regimen is frequently prescribed. At therapeutic serum levels (0.75–1.5 ng/mL) digoxin increases cardiac output and renal blood flow.

154. (E) Furosemide is a potent diuretic agent used to reduce the edema and excess sodium load. The sodium concentration is low in this patient because he has more excess fluid load than he has excess sodium load due to his CHF.

155. (A) A normal diet in the United States includes about 6–18 g sodium chloride daily. A restricted daily intake of 2–4 g would be recommended in a patient suffering from CHF with edema.

156. (E) About 60–90% of a digoxin dose is excreted unchanged by the kidneys. A decrease in kidney function (as monitored by BUN and serum creatinine) may necessitate a corresponding decrease in the daily digoxin dose. Hypokalemia, hypercalcemia, and hypomagnesemia may increase the potential for digoxin toxicity. Periodic electrolyte determinations are particularly important in patients receiving a diuretic or other drugs that may deplete potassium body stores.

157. (D) Most patients experience some digoxin toxicity at serum levels above 2 ng/mL. Following an oral dose of digoxin, there is a 6–8 h distributive phase. Plasma levels drawn during this time may be elevated. Analytical error and/or medication administration error must always be considered when examining a single laboratory value.

158. (B) A typical regimen for this patient would be 12.5 mg tid because the patient is already on furosemide and you do not want to induce volume depletion. In a patient not on a diuretic, the starting dose may be higher (25 mg tid).

159. (D) ACE inhibitors block the conversion of angiotensin I to angiotensin II, lessening the vasoconstrictive effects and causing venous and arterial vasodilation. ACE inhibitors have been shown to decrease long-term mortality in patients with CHF.

160. (D) Signs of digitalis toxicity include nausea, vomiting, bradycardia, ventricular and atrial arrhythmias, confusion, headaches, drowsiness, and visual disturbances such as photophobia and color aberrations.

161. (D) The inotropic and toxic effects of digoxin and calcium are synergistic. Fatal cardiac arrhythmias may result from IV administration of calcium in patients with digitalis toxicity.

162. (C) All three drugs interact with digoxin, but amiodarone and verapamil decrease systemic clearance and increase digoxin serum concentrations ranging from 35% to 104% with concurrent amiodarone therapy and up to 70% with verapamil therapy. Magnesium and aluminum salt antacids decrease GI absorption of digoxin, thus decreasing serum concentrations.

163. (A) All ACE inhibitors may produce a nonproductive persistent dry cough. Although manufacturers report an incidence of only 0.5–3%, published studies document much higher rates ranging from 5–25%. After discontinuation of the drug, the cough usually resolves within 1–4 days.

164. (A) Losartan is an angiotensin II receptor antagonist and also decreases afterload and preload via a mechanism similar to ACE inhibitors. Verapamil, diltiazem, and disopyramide are negative inotropic agents and would worsen heart failure in this patient. Clonidine is an effective agent for hypertension but does not affect afterload or preload.

165. (B) Typical initial losartan dosage regimens are 25 mg/d and may be increased to 50 mg/d.

166. (B) Losartan is not clinically affected by the administration of food and may be taken without regard to meals.

167. (A) Stat is the abbreviation for the Latin term *statim,* which is defined as "at once."

168. (D) Aspirin, TMP/SMX, rifampin, and metronidazole all interfere with warfarin kinetics either via absorption, metabolism, or protein binding.

169. (E) Warfarin interferes with the synthesis of vitamin K–dependent clotting factors II, VII, IX, and X.

170. (C) Warfarin takes approximately 1 week to see a maximum therapeutic effect. Heparin is needed for acute situations. Warfarin is a teratogen with an FDA pregnancy category of X and is contraindicated for use in pregnancy.

171. (B) Heparin has a direct inhibiting effect on clot formation via interaction with antithrombin III. Because its half-life is about 1 h at usual therapeutic doses, a heparin infusion will reach its steady state level in 5–7 h.

172. (C) A total of 4 mL of a concentrate heparin solution (5,000 units per mL) can be injected in a 500 mL bag of 5% dextrose for a final concentration of 20,000 units/500 mL.

173. (B) At a concentration of 20,000 units/500 mL, each milliliter contains 40 units of heparin. Thus, 25 mL of this admixture would be equivalent to 1,000 units of heparin. The final recommended rate would be 25 mL/h.

174. (C) The most common recommendations for PT ratios has been 1.5–3.5 times the laboratory control value. Because of some problems with standardization of this test, the World Health Organization (WHO) has promoted the use of international normalized ratio (INR).

175. (B) INR is defined as international normalized ratio and calculated as follows:

$$INR = (observed\ PT\ ratio)^{ISI}$$

ISI is the international sensitivity index, calibrated based on the type of thromboplastin used.

176. (D) For the treatment of pulmonary embolism and DVT an INR of 2.0–3.0 is recommended.

177. (E) All these points should be discussed with Ms. Colella. Compliance with warfarin is particularly important to maintain effective anticoagulation and prevent toxicity. All patients should be instructed to watch for bruising, bleeding gums, and other early signs of bleeding problems. Avoidance of drug interactions with warfarin is essential in preventing toxicity or subtherapeutic effects. Patients should be instructed to contact their pharmacist or physician before stopping or starting any new medication, particularly OTC products.

178. (C) During the first 4 weeks after discharge, weekly monitoring is usually required. However, once the patient has attained an effective anticoagulation state and maintains a stable diet and other drug regimens, monthly laboratory monitoring is adequate.

179. (D) *P aeruginosa* is the most common bacterial pathogen isolated from the sputum of cystic fibrosis patients followed by *S aureus* and *H influenzae*.

180. (A) The sweat test is most commonly used for the diagnosis although chromosomal analysis is also available.

181. (A) Pancrease contains lipase, protease, and amylase. However, when substituting products, it is the lipase portion that should be compared to get an equivalent dose.

182. (D) Pancreatic enzymes are readily destroyed by gastric acid. When ranitidine is used to increase the pH of the stomach and upper small intestinal tract, less of the pancrease is destroyed and therefore, smaller doses can be used.

183. (E) Cystic fibrosis patients may be deficient in all of the fat soluble vitamins if a lack of pancreatic enzymes leads to steatorrhea and fat malabsorption.

184. (D) If the deficiency is severe enough that treatment is warranted, phytonadione (vitamin K) can be administered.

185. (E) All of the above.

186. (D) Ganciclovir, foscarnet, and cidofovir are antivirals approved for the treatment of CMV retinitis.

187. (D)   If sputum does not contain cysts, a lavage is done and biopsy of lung tissue is best.

188. (B)   *P carinii* pneumonia is a pulmonary disease caused by a protozoan parasite usually dormant in the host lung, but activated in an immunocompromised host (i.e., HIV positive, cancer chemotherapy). The mortality rate of *P carinii* pneumonitis in such compromised patients is 90–100% if no specific treatment is given. *P carinii* has two forms: (1) cystic thick-walled and spherical, which can contain up to eight sporozoites (intracellular cysts), and (2) extracystic or trephozoites, thin-walled with indefinite cell membranes. These cells invade alveoli walls, attaching to macrophages, PMNs, and peritoneal tissue.

189. (E)   Psoriasis is a skin condition of accelerated skin cell turnover, characterized by tough silvery scales over an inflamed area of the skin. It is often chronic and may require aggressive methods to slow down cell turnover.

190. (E)   All of these products are in FDA Pregnancy Category X.

191. (D)   Selegiline and benzotropine are both agents used as adjunctive therapy in the treatment of parkinsonism. Vercuronium bromide is a neuromuscular blocking agent administered parenterally during surgery to produce skeletal muscle relaxation.

192. (E)   Patients with warts in any of these areas should be referred to a physician.

193. (E)   All of these products require loading doses for most effective therapy.

194. (E)   Alcohol can cause an untoward reaction when combined with any of these products.

195. (E)   All of the listed products require a test dose prior to the initiation of therapy.

196. (C)   Approximately 95% of ethanol is oxidized in the liver. The remaining 5% is excreted through the lungs and kidneys.

197. (B)   Enzyme induction increases the amount of enzyme in the liver, thereby increasing the rate of drug metabolism.

198. (C)   Acute ethanol administration inhibits both phase I and phase II biotransformation.

199. (B)   Absolute bioavailability refers to the rate and extent of system absorption of a drug administered from an extravascular dosage form as compared to the amount of drug available after IV administration.

200. (B)   Quinidine gluconate and quinidine sulfate are different salts. Chemical or pharmaceutical equivalents must contain the same active ingredient.

201. (D)   Oral administration of propranolol, verapamil, lidocaine, morphine, and nitroglycerin results in significant metabolism by the liver before the drug reaches the systemic circulation.

202. (E)   Phenobarbital is a weak acid (pKa 7.2). Renal clearance increases with alkalinization of the urine. Amphetamine is a weak base; acidification of the urine increases renal excretion of amphetamine.

203. (D)   Acetylcysteine can be used to decrease acetaminophen-induced hepatotoxicity as well as a mucolytic to decrease the viscosity of lung secretions in patients with cystic fibrosis.

204. (B)   Common adverse reactions to anticholinergics are due to reduction of the volume of salivary and other GI fluid secretions, prolonged inhibition of GI motility, decreased contractility of the bladder, and decreased ocular accommodation. Atropine and other anticholinergic agents are potent bronchodilators.

205. (C)   It takes approximately 4–7 half-lives for a drug that exhibits first-order pharmacokinetics to reach steady state. This correlates well for nortriptyline with the clinical findings that it often takes up to 2 weeks to observe maximum effect.

206. (B)   Fluoride has a dual mode of action: it inhibits bacterial reproduction and strengthens tooth enamel.

207. (E)   The primary ingredient of Primatene Mist Inhaler is epinephrine. Patients with the listed conditions should only use inhaled epinephrine under the advice of a physician.

208. (C)   Hormones do not possess cytotoxic activity, but are effective against tumors in hormone-response tissue (e.g., breast, endometrium).

209. (A)   Although some chemotherapeutic agents have only a "minor" effect on bone marrow, most antineoplastic drugs do depress the bone marrow, and this must be considered when determining the maximum dose.

210. (C)   Aminobenzoic acid (formerly known as para-aminobenzoic acid) is used in many sunscreen products in concentrations up to 15%.

211. (E)   Quinidine prolongs the refractory period. It has a narrow therapeutic range and toxicity can cause cardiac arrest. GI symptoms occur in approximately 30% of patients and may warrant discontinuation of the drug.

212. (B)   β-Adrenergic drugs reduce sympathetic stimulation at the heart to slow the heart rate and decrease myocardial oxygen demand.

213. (D)   SSRIs have been shown to be more effective in treating panic disorders but are significantly more expensive than some of the older traditional therapies.

214. (E) Angina, or transient chest discomfort, is caused by insufficient myocardial oxygen. All of these conditions affect oxygen supply to this tissue.

215. (D) Rapid venous dilation produced by nitrates causes a pronounced vascular headache. Administration of acetaminophen 30 min before nitrate use may prevent or minimize the headache.

216. (E) Carbidopa is a decarboxylase inhibitor, which decreases the required dosage of levodopa. It has no therapeutic effect in parkinsonism when administered alone.

217. (B) Unlike other antacids, sodium bicarbonate can be significantly absorbed into the systemic circulation. Milk-alkali syndrome results from systemic alkalosis and large amounts of calcium in the gut.

218. (C) Rifampin may color sweat, tears, feces, and urine a bright orange-red. Rifampin may stain soft contact lenses.

219. (D) Clavulanic acid contains a β-lactam ring and an oxazolidine ring. It has only weak antibacterial activity alone, but produces a synergistic effect when combined with certain penicillins or cephalosporins.

220. (C) Dornase-alfa should be stored between 2 and 8° C.

221. (A) Concurrent administration of ascorbic acid may increase iron absorption. Antacids and meals often interfere with iron absorption. If nausea and vomiting from iron administration is not significant, recommend iron intake between meals.

222. (A) Iron dextran is available for parenteral administration only.

223. (C) The adult male and postmenopausal female require a daily iron intake of 10–12 mg. Menstruating women and pregnant women require 18 mg.

224. **(B)** Iron administration is contraindicated in patients with hemochromatosis, a syndrome characterized by excessive iron stores, causing skin pigmentation and pancreatic damage. Transfused red blood cells often contain significant amounts of iron.

225. **(B)** Constant thirst is a common symptom of diabetes. Fatigue is the most common symptom of iron deficiency.

226. **(E)** Only a few cases are secondary and are generally caused by drugs such as dopamine antagonists or chemicals such as carbon monoxide.

227. **(A)** Pill-rolling or bread-crumbling hand movements, muscle rigidity, blank facial stare, drooling, and slurred speech are all symptomatic of parkinsonism.

228. **(E)** Increasing the amount or duration of dopamine or suppressing acetylcholine ameliorates the symptoms of parkinsonism.

229. **(C)** Anticholinergic effects include dry mouth, constipation, urinary retention, loss of memory, and decreased gastric function.

230. **(B)** Decreased levodopa activity may be produced as a result of delayed gastric emptying when used in combination with anticholinergics.

231. **(A)** APTT is the most sensitive indicator of bleeding and clotting.

232. **(D)** Carbidopa inhibits peripheral decarboxylation of levodopa. The combination contains carbidopa:levodopa in a ratio of 1:10, and generally produces fewer GI side effects.

233. **(A)** Bromocriptine may produce cardiovascular collapse, hypotension, drowsiness, GI upset, and hallucinations.

234. **(D)** A drug holiday with titrated reintroduction of drugs generally decreases side effects and reduces the dosage

required to control symptoms. The patient will likely have fewer on–off episodes.

235. **(E)** Lack of response from an antibiotic can stem from a variety of causes, as listed. The situation needs to be reassessed before altering the regimen.

236. **(C)** Alprazolam is considered a shorter acting benzodiazepine when compared to clonazepam and diazepam.

237. **(E)** All of the listed drugs have been associated with the development of Stevens-Johnson syndrome, a potentially fatal complication.

238. **(E)** The procaine and benzathine forms of penicillin are insoluble and allow slow drug absorption following intramuscular injection.

239. **(E)** Headaches are the most common side effect of nitroglycerin therapy; dosage reduction may be necessary if headaches persist. Dermatitis also often accompanies transdermal therapy; rotating application sites minimizes this reaction.

240. **(A)** The usual initial dosing range for transdermal nitroglycerin is 5–15 mg/24 h. These doses represent the expected release rate from the patches, not the actual nitroglycerin content of the dosage form (i.e., a 15 mg/24 h delivered dose may actually be obtained from a transdermal system that contains 120 mg nitroglycerin).

241. **(D)** Nitroglycerin relaxes vascular smooth muscle, thereby reducing myocardial oxygen consumption.

242. **(B)** Flecainide is an antiarrhythmic agent used to treat ventricular arrhythmias. Beta blockers and nitrates reduce myocardial oxygen demands, whereas calcium channel blockers enhance myocardial oxygen supply.

243. **(A)** Patients experiencing myocardial infarction usually have severe chest pain that may radiate to the left arm, neck,

and jaw. Muscle aches and frequent urination at night are not considered common signs of a myocardial infarction.

244. (A) The smaller the number, the larger the diameter of the needle.

245. (E) All of the listed conditions may contribute to the development of digoxin toxicity.

246. (D) High concentrations of quinidine have been associated with cinchonism. Symptoms include blurred vision, headache, tinnitus, nausea, and mental changes.

247. (B) Patients on digoxin are predisposed to digoxin toxicity if potassium levels are too low.

248. (E) All of the listed conditions are considered predisposing factors for developing pulmonary tuberculosis.

249. (D) Combinations of chemotherapeutic agents are usually used in the treatment of leukemias and lymphomas because of superior cell kill rates.

250. (A) Alkylating agents, such as nitrogen mustard, severely depress bone marrow, with the nadir observed 8–10 days after administration.

251. (A) NSAIDs can significantly increase methotrexate blood levels. The proposed mechanism of action involves inhibition of both the glomerular filtration and renal secretion of methotrexate.

252. (C) Methotrexate may be administered as a single 7.5-mg dose once weekly or as three 2.5-mg doses at 12-h intervals each week. Total weekly dose should not exceed 20 mg.

253. (D) Methotrexate is used for the management of severe rheumatoid arthritis. Response to therapy is not immediate; a minimum of 3 weeks is usually required to observe any measurable improvement in symptoms.

254. (E) The bioavailability of oral methotrexate is dose-dependent and may be affected by food intake, nonabsorbable antibiotics, and a shortened intestinal transit time. The bioavailability may be as low as 20% at higher doses.

255. (D) As an antidote to a methotrexate medication error, leucovorin should be administered IV or IM in an amount equal to the weight of methotrexate.

256. (B) Cyclophosphamide and nitrogen mustard are alkylating agents that interfere with DNA replication.

257. (B) The major side effects of doxorubicin are hematologic and cardiovascular. Hemorrhagic cystitis occurs frequently in patients receiving cyclophosphamide.

258. (B) Seborrhea is generally found in areas associated with hair and oil glands; thus, the scalp is a primary site of the condition. Medicated shampoos comprise the majority of treatment modes.

259. (D) Reducing cell turnover while removing existing scales should bring the psoriatic episode under control.

260. (E) Fungi and yeast grow best on moist, dark, warm sites on the skin, and are particularly seen when the patient is immunosuppressed or has been on broad-spectrum antibiotics.

261. (C) Pyoderma is a skin condition in which pus is present. This is characteristic of a bacterial infection.

262. (C) Tinea corporis is a fungal infection of the skin that often spreads in a circular lesion.

263. (E) Triptorelin, a luteinizing hormone-releasing hormone (LHRH) agonist, was approved by the FDA in 2000 for the treatment of advanced prostate cancer

264. (A) Gemtuzumab, a recombinant humanized anti-CD33 monoclonal antibody and cytotoxic antitumor antibiotic, was approved by the FDA in 2000 for the treatment of acute myeloid leukemia.

265. (B) Capecitabine, an oral prodrug of both doxifluridine and 5-fluorouracil, was approved by the FDA in 1998 for the treatment of metastatic breast cancer.

266. (C) Valrubicin, an anthracycline (doxorubicin analog), was approved by the FDA in 1998 for the treatment of bladder cancer (carcinoma in situ).

267. (D) Temozolomide, an alkylating antineoplastic agent, was approved by the FDA in 1999 for the treatment of refractory astrocytoma.

268. (B) Imatinib, a selective tyrosine kinase inhibitor, was approved by the FDA in 2001 for the treatment of chronic myelogenous leukemia.

269. (C) Alitretinoin, a naturally occurring endogenous retinoid with actions similar to all-trans-retinoic acid (tretinoin), was approved by the FDA in 1999 for the treatment of cutaneous lesions associated with Kaposi sarcoma.

270. (B) Toremifene, an antiestrogen agent chemically related to tamoxifen, has been effective in the treatment of advanced breast cancer.

271. (B) Citalopram, a selective serotonin reuptake inhibitor, was FDA approved in 1998 for the treatment of depression.

272. (B) Rivastigamine, a carbamate acetylcholinesterase inhibitor with regional selectivity for the hippocampus, was FDA approved in 2000 for the treatment of dementia associated with mild to moderate Alzheimer's disease.

273. (C) Ziprasidone, an atypical antipyschotic agent, was approved by the FDA in 2001, for the treatment of schizophrenia.

274. (D) Oxcarbazepine, an antiepileptic drug derived from carbamazepine, was FDA approved in 2000 for the treatment of partial seizures in children (>4 y) and adults.

275. (E) Levetiracetam is a broad-spectrum antiepileptic agent approved by the FDA in 1999 for the treatment of partial seizures in adults.

276. (E) Cefditoren was approved by the FDA in 2001 for the treatment of acute bacterial exacerbation of chronic bronchitis, pharyngitis/tonsillitis, and uncomplicated skin and skin structure infections.

277. (C) Dalfopristin/quinupristin, the first water-soluble streptogramin antibiotic combination for IV administration, was approved by the FDA in 1999 for the treatment of vancomycin-resistant *Enterococcus faecium,* as well as for treatment of complicated skin and skin structure infections caused by *S aureus*.

278. (D) Rifapentine, an antibacterial, was approved by the FDA in 1998 for the treatment of tuberculosis infections.

279. (B) Formivirsen, an antisene compound, was approved by the FDA in 1998 as an intravitreal injection for the treatment of CMV retinitis.

280. (B) Amprenavir, a protease inhibitor, was FDA approved in 1999 for the treatment of HIV infection.

281. (B) Argatroban, a selective thrombin inhibitor, was approved by the FDA in 2000 as an anticoagulant in hemodialysis patients.

282. (D) Nesiritide was approved by the FDA in August 2001 for the IV treatment of patients with acutely decompensated CHF who have dyspnea at rest or with minimal activity.

283. (B) Candesartan, an angiotensin II receptor antagonist, was approved by the FDA in 1998 for the treatment of hypertension.

284. (C) Dofetilide, a pure class III antiarrhythmic agent, was approved by the FDA in 1999 for the maintenance of normal sinus rhythm (delay in time to recurrence of atrial fibrillation/atrial flutter [AF/AFl]) in patients with AF/AFI of >1 week duration who have been converted to normal sinus rhythm.

285. (E) Tirofiban, an antiplatelet agent that binds to the platelet receptor glycoprotein IIb/IIIa and inhibits platelet aggregation, was approved by the FDA in 1998 for the treatment of acute coronary syndromes.

286. (B) Sirolimus solution was FDA approved in 1999 as an immunosuppressant for organ transplant recipients.

287. (C) Montelukast, a leukotriene receptor antagonist, was approved by the FDA in 1998 for the treatment of asthma.

288. (E) Formoterol was approved by the FDA in September 2001 for the long-term, twice-daily (morning and evening) administration in the maintenance treatment of bronchoconstriction in patients with COPD including chronic bronchitis and emphysema.

289. (D) Rofecoxib, a COX-2 inhibitor, was approved by the FDA in 1999 for the treatment of dysmenorrhea, osteoarthritis, and acute pain.

290. (B) Brinzolamide, a topical ophthalmic carbonic anhydrase inhibitor, was approved by the FDA in 1998 for the treatment of open angle glaucoma.

291. (B) Nitric oxide was approved in December 1999 for the treatment of term and near-term (>34 weeks) neonates with hypoxic respiratory failure associated with clinical or echocardiographic evidence of pulmonary hypertension, where it improves oxygenation and reduces the need for extracorporeal membrane oxygenation.

292. (A) Zaleplon was approved in August 1999 for the short-term treatment of insomnia.

293. (C) Entacapone was approved in October 1999 as an adjunct to levodopa/carbidopa to treat patients with idiopathic Parkinson's disease who experience the signs and symptoms of end-of-dose "wearing-off" (so-called "fluctuating" patients).

294. (D) Rizatriptan, a 5HT-1 receptor agonist, was approved in 1998 for the treatment of acute migraines.

295. (E) Exemestane was approved by the FDA in October 1999 for the treatment of advanced breast cancer in postmenopausal women whose disease has progressed following tamoxifen therapy.

296. (B) Galantamine, a selective, long-acting, acetylcholinesterase inhibitor, was approved in June 2001 for the treatment of mild to moderate dementia of the Alzheimer's type.

297. (D) Vanganciclovir, a prodrug (valyl ester) of ganciclovir, was approved for the treatment of CMV retinitis in patients with AIDS.

298. (C) Oral budenoside was FDA approved in October 2001 for the treatment of mild to moderate active Crohn's disease involving the ileum and/or ascending colon.

299. (B) Almotriptan, a 5HT-1 receptor agonist, was approved in 2001 for the treatment of acute migraines.

300. (E) Esomperazole, a proton pump inhibitor, was approved in 2001 for the treatment of erosive esophagitis.

References

Briggs G, Freeman RK, Yaffe SJ (Eds.): *Drugs in Pregnancy and Lactation,* 5th Ed., Baltimore, MD: Williams & Wilkins, 1998.

Berardi RR, Allen LV, DeSimone EM (Eds.): *Handbook of Nonprescription Drugs,* 12th Ed., Washington, DC: American Pharmaceutical Association, 2000.

DiPiro JT, Schwinghammer TL, Wells B (Eds.): *Pharmacotherapy: A Pathophysiologic Approach,* 4th Ed., Stamford, CT: Appleton & Lange, 1999.

Gennaro AR, et al. (Eds.): *Remington's The Science and Practice of Pharmacy,* 19th Ed., Easton, PA: Mack Publishers, 1995.

Grabenstein JD: *Immunofacts: Vaccines and Immunologic Drugs,* St. Louis, MO: Drug Facts and Comparisons, 1995.

Hansten PD, Horn JR (Eds.): *Drug Interactions: Analysis and Management,* St. Louis, MO: Drug Facts and Comparisons, 2001.

Hardman JG, Limbird LE (Eds.): *Goodman & Gilman's Pharmcological Basis of Therapeutics,* 9th Ed., New York, NY: McGraw Hill, 1996.

Malone PM, Mosdell KW, Kier KL, Stanovich JE: *Drug Information: A Guide for Pharmacists,* Stamford, CT: Appleton & Lange, 1996.

Olin BR (Ed.): *Drug Facts and Comparisons,* St. Louis, MO: Facts and Comparisons, 2001.

Shargel L and Yu A: *Applied Biopharmaceutics and Pharmacokinetics,* 3rd Ed., Norwalk, CT: Appleton & Lange, 1993.

Siberry GK: *The Harriet Lane Handbook,* 15th Ed., St. Louis, MO: Mosby Year Book Inc., 2000.

Taketomo CK, Hodding JH, Kraus DM (Eds.): *APhA Pediatric Dosage Handbook 2001–2002,* Hudson, OH: Lexicomp Inc., 2001

Tatro DS. *Drug Interaction Facts,* St. Louis, MO: Facts and Comparisons, 2001.

Traub SL (Ed.): *Basic Skills in Interpreting Laboratory Data,* Bethesda, MD: American Society of Hospitals, 1996.

Winters ME: *Basic Clinical Pharmacokinetics,* 3rd Ed., Vancouver, WA: Applied Therapeutics Inc., 1994.

Appendix

Table A–1. FDA Approved Drugs: January 2000 through October 2001

Generic Name	Brand Name	Company Name	Indication	Dosage Form	FDA	Pharm Class	Year
	Trinam	Eurogene Ltd	Prevention of intimal hyperplasia	Other	Orphan	Gene-based therapy	2000
	ABX-CBL	Abgenix Inc	Steroid resistant graft vs host disease	Parenteral	Orphan	Monoclonal antibody	2000
Almotriptan	Axert	Pharmacia/Upjohn	Acute migraine treatment	Oral	1S	Serotonin-1 receptor agonist	2001
Alosetron[a]	Lotronex	Glaxo Wellcome	Irritable bowel syndrome in women	Oral	1S	Selective serotonin antagonist	2000
Argatroban	Acova	Texas Biotech	Anticoagulant in hemodialysis patients	Parenteral	1S	Selective thrombin inhibitor	2000
Arsenic Trioxide	Trisenox	Cell Therapeutics	Treatment of APL	Parenteral	1PV	Antineoplastic arsenical cmpd.	2000
Articaine HCl 4%	Septocaine	Deproco	Local anesthesia	Parenteral	1S	Local amide type anesthetic	2000
Atovaquone/Proguanil	Malarone	Glaxo Wellcome	Malaria	Oral	3S	Antimicrobials	2000
Balsalazide	Colazal	Salix Pharmaceuticals	Mild to moderate active ulcerative colitis	Oral	1S	Prodrug of mesalamine	2000
Bimatoprost	Lumigan	Allergan	Ocular hypertension	Ophthalmic	1P	Prostamide analogue	2001
Bivalirudin	Angiomax	Medicines Co	Prevention of clotting in angina/PTCA	Parenteral	1S	Anticoagulant	2000
Botulinum Toxin Type B	Myobloc	Elan Corp	Cervical dystonia	Parenteral	2S	Miscellaneous	2000
Budesonide	Entocort EC	Astra Zeneca LP	Mild to moderate active Crohn's disease	Oral	3P	Glucocorticoid	2001
Caspofungin acetate	Cancidas	Merck Research	Refractory aspergillosis infections	Parenteral	1P	Antifungal	2001
Cefditoren pivoxil	Spectracef	TAP Pharmaceuticals	Acute bacterial infections	Oral	1S	Cephalosporin anti-infective	2001

324

Cetrorelix Acetate	Cetrotide	Asta Medica	Prevention of premature LH surges	Parenteral	1S	LHRH antagonist	2000
Cetrotide	Cetrorelix	Astra Medica	Prevention of premature LH surges	Parenteral	1S	Miscellaneous	2000
Cevimeline	Evoxac	Snowbrand	Xerostomia with Sjörgen's syndrome	Oral	1S	Muscarinic agonist	2000
Colesevelam	Welchol	Gel Tex	Reduction of LDLs	Oral	1S	Bile acid sequestrant	2000
Docosanol	Abreva	Avanir Pharmaceutical	Treatment of cold sore/fever blister	Topical	1S	Anti-viral agent	2000
Drospirenone/Ethinyl	Yasmin	Berlex Labs	Contraception	Oral	1, 4S	Contraception	2001
Ethinyl	Nuvaring	Organon Inc	Contraception	Vaginal sponge	1S	Contraceptive	2001
Fluticasone/Salmeterol	Advair Diskus	Glaxo Wellcome	Asthma (maintenance)	Inhalation		Antiasthma agents	2000
Formoterol	Foradil	Novartis Pharmaceuticals	Asthma (maintenance treatment)	Inhalation	1S	Beta-2 agonist	2001
Galantamine	Reminyl	Janssen Research Fdn	Mild to moderate dementia in Alzheimer's	Oral	1S	Acetylcholinesterase inhibitor	2001
Gemtuzumab Ozogamicin	Mylotarg	Wyeth Ayerst	Refactory or relapsed CD33+ AML	Parenteral	1PV	Cytotoxic antibiotic	2000
Imatinib	Gleevec	Novartis Pharmaceuticals	Chronic myeloid leukemia	Oral	1P, V	Antineoplastic	2001
Insulin Aspart	NovoLog	Novo Nordisk	Adult patients with diabetes mellitus	Subcutaneous/IM	1S	Rapid acting insulin analog	2000
Insulin Glargine	Lantus	Aventis	Type 1 and type 2 diabetes mellitus	Subcutaneous/IM	1S	Long acting recombinant insulin	2000
Linezolid	Zyvox	Pharmacia and Upjohn	Antibiotic resistant gram (+) cocci	Oral	1P	Oxaxolidinone antibiotic	2000
Lopinavir	Kaletra	Abbott Labs	HIV infection	Oral	1S	Antiviral	2000
Lopinavir; Ritonavir	Kaletra	Abbott Labs	Treatment of HIV infection	Oral	1, 4P	HIV protease inhibitor	2000
Meloxicam	Mobic	Boehringer Pharmaceuticals	Osteoarthritis	Oral	1S	Nonsteroidal Antiinflammatory	2000
Mesalamine	Canasa	Axcan Scandipharm Inc	Active ulcerative proctitis	Rectal	5P	5-ASA	2001
Mifepristone	Mifeprex	Population Council	Abortifacient	Oral	1P	Progesterone receptor antag.	2000
Natglinide	Starlix	Novartis	Type II diabetes	Oral	1S	Hypoglycemic	2000

Table A–1. (*cont.*)

Generic Name	Brand Name	Company Name	Indication	Dosage Form	FDA	Pharm Class	Year
Nesiritide citrate	Natrecor	Scios Inc	Acutely decompensated CHF	Parenteral	1S	Cardiac hormone	2001
Oxacarbazepine	Trileptal	Novartis Pharmaceuticals	Partial seizures in epileptic children, 4–16 y	Oral	1S	Antiepileptic	2000
Pantoprazole Sodium	Protonix	Wyeth Ayerst	Short-term treatment of erosive esophagitis	Oral	1S	Proton pump inhibitor	2000
Perfultren	Definity	Dupont Pharmaceuticals	Diagnostic aid used in echocardiograms	Parenteral	1S	Contrast dye	2001
Rivastigmine Tartrate	Exelon	Novartis Pharmaceuticals	Mild to moderate dementia of Alzheimer's type	Oral	1S	Carbamate Ach inhibitor	2000
SERPACWA[b]	SERPACWA	US Army	Reduce or delay absorption through skin	Topical	1P	Reduce/delay skin absorption	2000
Tinzaparin Sodium	Innohep	Dupont Pharmaceuticals	Acute symptomatic deep vein thrombosis	Parenteral	1S	Low molecular weight Heparin	2000
Travoprost	Travatan	Alcon Universal	Open angle glaucoma/ocular hypertension	Ophthalmic	1P	Prostaglandin F2-alpha analogue	2001
Triptorelin	Trelstar	Debio Recherchie Pharm	Advanced prostate cancer (pallative care)	Injection	3S	Antineoplastic	2001
Triptorelin Pamoate	Trelstar Depot	Debio Recherche	Advanced prostate cancer	Parenteral	1S	LHRH agonist	2000
Unoprostone Isopropyl	Rescula	Ciba Vision	Lower pressure in open angle glaucoma	Topical	1P	Prostaglandin F2-alpha analog	2000
Valganciclovir	Valcyte	Sytnex Inc	Cytomegalovirus (CMV) retinitis in AIDS	Oral	2P	Anti-viral agent	2001
Verteporfin	Visudyne	QLT Photo Therapeutics	Age-related macular degeneration	Parenteral	1P	Photosensitizing agent	2000

Ziprasidone	Geodon	Pfizer Labs	Schizophrenia	Oral	1S	Atypical antipsychotic	2001
Zoledronic acid	Zometa	Novartis Pharmaceuticals	Hypercalcemia of malignancy	Parenteral	1P	Bisphosphonate	2001
Zonisamide	Zonegran	Elan Pharmaceuticals	Adjunct therapy of partial seizures in adults	Oral	1S	Broad spectrum anticonvulsant	2000

[a]Alosetron was withdrawn from the US market in November 2000 (see *http://www.fda.gov/bbs/topics/ANSWERS/ANS01058.html*).

[b]Skin Exposure Reduction Paste Against Chemical Warfare Agents.

FDA Ratings: Chemical status; 1 = new chemical entity, 2 = new salt form, 3 = new dosage form, 4 = new combination, 5 = already marketed drug product but a new manufacturer

Therapeutic Status: P = priority, therapeutic advantage, provides improved treatment of modest advantage when compared to marketed drugs, S = standard, similar therapeutic properties over marketed drugs, V = orphan drug.